www.ha[...]ional.com

Bringing you [...] Health Sciences
companies including Baillière Tindall, Churchill Livingstone,
Mosby and W.B. Saunders

- **Browse** for latest information on new books, journals and electronic products

- **Search** for information on over 20 000 published titles with full product information including tables of contents and sample chapters

- **Keep up to date** with our extensive publishing programme in your field by registering with **eAlert** or requesting postal updates

- **Secure online ordering** with prompt delivery, as well as full contact details to order by phone, fax or post

- **News** of special features and promotions

If you are based in the following countries, please visit the country-specific site to receive full details of product availability and local ordering information

USA: www.harcourthealth.com

Canada: www.harcourtcanada.com

Australia: www.harcourt.com.au

Baillière Tindall   CHURCHILL LIVINGSTONE   Mosby   W.B. SAUNDERS

Notes for the DRCOG

Commissioning Editor: Ellen Green
Project Development Manager: Siân Jarman
Project Manager: Nancy Arnott
Designer: Erik Bigland

Notes for the DRCOG

Jo Anthony
MA MB BChir FRCOG

Consultant in Obstetrics and Gynaecology
Northampton General Hospital

Peter Kaye
MA MB FRCP MRCGP DRCOG

Consultant in Palliative Medicine
Cynthia Spencer House, Northampton

FOURTH EDITION

CHURCHILL
LIVINGSTONE

EDINBURGH LONDON NEW YORK PHILADELPHIA ST LOUIS SYDNEY
TORONTO 2001

CHURCHILL LIVINGSTONE
An imprint of Harcourt Publishers Limited

© Harcourt Publishers Limited 2001

First published 1983
Second edition 1988
Third edition 1995
Fourth edition 2001

ISBN 0-443-06418-0

British Library Cataloguing in Publication Data
A catalogue record for this book is available from the British
Library

Library of Congress Cataloging in Publication Data
A catalog record for this book is available from the Library of
Congress

Note
Medical knowledge is constantly changing. As new information
becomes available, changes in treatment, procedures, equipment
and the use of drugs become necessary. The authors and the
publishers have taken care to ensure that the information given in
this text is accurate and up to date. However, readers are strongly
advised to confirm that the information, especially with regard to
drug usage, complies with the latest legislation and standards of
practice.

The
publisher's
policy is to use
paper manufactured
from sustainable forests

Printed in China

Preface to the fourth edition

This is now the fourth edition of a book which started out as revision notes written by a GP in training, but which has evolved into a complete textbook on the subject.

I sometimes think that writing a book is the male equivalent to having a baby, with the gestation of ideas, the painful labour of writing, the delivery of the manuscript (the publisher being the midwife!) and the arrival of a book which, if it is healthy, will grow and develop with time. The 'growth' of this book into a new edition brings me great joy, but its development has only been possible with the help of others (all female!).

Most importantly, this book has developed as a result of the involvement and expertise of Jo Anthony, a Consultant in Obstetrics and Gynaecology, and a gold medal winner in the MRCOG examination. A busy clinician and teacher, she is an excellent lecturer and writer and is now an examiner for the DRCOG. This means that the book is authoritative, up to date and clinically relevant, but still short enough to be an excellent revision text. The book has been carefully checked throughout to bring it up to date, with several parts rewritten, and we have also enlarged the chapter on the structure and regulations of the DRCOG to include some very useful practical advice.

Once again we are very grateful to Fran Ackland (Consultant Paediatrician at Northampton General Hospital) for her expert comments on the chapter on the neonate, and to Betty Verney (Senior Midwife at Northampton General Hospital) for her helpful comments on the section on Obstetrics. We would also like to thank Siân Jarman, the Project Development Manager at Harcourt Health Sciences, for her support and encouragement.

We hope this book continues to be useful to both SHOs in training, GPs and medical students.

Northampton 2001   P.K.

Contents

4. Obstetrics 100

5. The neonate 185

6. The DRCOG exam 208

1. Gynaecology

Gynaecology is but one part of general medicine and overall health. The symptoms and signs must always be interpreted as a part of the *whole* – the choice of treatment will vary between individuals and at different times in the same individual.

◆ History: Key points

1. *The specific complaint* – if multiple check the order of importance to the patient: this leads to a more stepwise approach to sorting out complex or multiple symptoms and therapeutic decisions.
2. *Date of LMP* and cycle (e.g. 5/28, regular or irregular?).
   - period pains (during or preceding the bleeding? analgesia used?)
   - heaviness (clots? flooding? use of both towels and tampons?)
   - other bleeding (intermenstrual, postcoital)
   - age of menarche
   - any episodes of amenorrhoea?
3. *Parity* – detailed obstetric history: terminations/ectopics/ miscarriages.
4. *Discharge* (colour, duration, itch, soreness, partner).
5. *Abdomen* (pain, bowels, dysuria, stress or urge incontinence).
6. *Intercourse* (pain, problems, libido).
7. *Contraception.*
8. *Drugs* (particularly O/C or HRT).
9. *Past history* – date of last smear, previous gynae surgery (curettage, colposcopy/cautery/cone biopsy, laparoscopy), general surgery, medical conditions.
10. *Emotional problems/stress* (marital and family/work/social).

◆ Examination: Relevant findings

1. *General appearance* (weight and height, breasts, hirsutism).
2. Palpate the *abdomen* (laparoscopy scars, tenderness, lumps).
3. Inspect the *vulva* (redness, atrophy, urethral discharge, Bartholin's cysts, warts, ulceration or carcinoma).
4. Pass a speculum, inspect the *cervix* and take a smear if required (see colposcopy section). Take a *high vaginal swab* (HVS) including chlamydia, gonococcus if appropriate (urethral and endocervical), trichomonas. Immediate microscopy and pH can be helpful. Be familiar with both the Cuscoe and Sims specula and their appropriate usage.
5. *Bimanual examination.* Tenderness on moving the cervix occurs in salpingitis and ectopic pregnancy. Note whether the os is small and nulliparous or patulous and multiparous. Note whether the

uterus is anteverted, axial or retroverted and whether it is enlarged (pregnancy or fibroids). Palpate the adnexae for tenderness or lumps (when ultrasound and/or laparoscopy may be necessary for diagnosis). Rectal examination if appropriate.

◆ Physiology of the normal menstrual cycle

1. *Bleeding* occurs because corpus luteal function fades, oestrogen and progesterone levels fall (and FSH rises) and the unsupported endometrium sloughs. The average blood loss is approximately 60 ml and clotting is prevented by endometrial fibrinolysins. Passing clots reflects heavy loss which exceeds the normal fibrinolytic capacity of the uterus.

2. The rising FSH from the pituitary stimulates follicular development (*follicular phase*): usually only one follicle is selected for maximum growth that cycle but all follicles involved in that cycle can secrete oestrogen. Oestrogen causes duct proliferation in the breast and glandular changes in the endometrium (*proliferative phase*) and increases and modifies the cervical mucus. Important structural changes occur in the mucus under the influence of oestrogen (favourable mucus: good postcoital test results).

3. The rising oestrogen causes (positive feedback) an LH surge, precipitating ovulation of the dominant follicle.

4. The corpus luteum formed thereafter secretes progesterone (*luteal phase*). Changes include an elevation in temperature (0.5°C), secretory changes in the breast ducts and endometrium (secretory type on histology) and unfavourable cervical mucus.

5. *Implantation* of a fertilised ovum results in HCG secretion by the trophoblast. This has an LH-like action and supports the corpus luteum, which continues to secrete oestrogen and progesterone, maintaining the endometrium until the placenta takes over (12 weeks).

   Ovulation can be demonstrated by:
   - ovulatory cascade of cervical mucus (Billing's method)
   - raised body temperature (+0.25–0.5°C)
   - raised serum progesterone on day 21. Urinary hormones change but are no longer measured clinically
   - endometrial biopsy (shows secretory changes in the luteal phase of the cycle)
   - ultrasound (follicle not seen, fluid in POD)

◆ Oestrogens

Oestradiol 17β is synthesised from cholesterol and metabolised to oestrone and oestriol. They are excreted in the urine and can be measured (e.g. during FSH therapy). Synthetic preparations are used therapeutically (ethinyloestradiol and, less commonly, stilboestrol). Premarin is a mixture of conjugated oestrogens derived from pregnant mares' urine. Oestrogens have the following *actions*:
- pituitary inhibition
- secondary sexual development
- fusion of the epiphyses
- myometrial hypertrophy

- endometrial hyperplasia (hence withdrawal bleeds when used in opposed HRT or combined contraceptive pills)
- increased 'favourable' cervical mucus
- vaginal cornification (increased squames)
- sodium retention
- tendency to thrombosis

They are *used* in:

1. The combined pill.
2. Hormone replacement therapy: after the menopause, for atrophic vaginitis or hot flushes, or in ovarian dysgenesis/Turner's syndrome patients (e.g. ethinyloestradiol 20–50 μg daily). Prolonged use of unopposed oestrogens causes endometrial hyperplasia or even malignancy (oppose with cyclical progestogens at least days 12–28 to counteract this).
3. Atrophic vaginitis pre-puberty: with caution.
4. Cancer: Stilboestrol is less potent than ethinyloestradiol and is used to treat carcinoma of the prostate (1 mg daily). Now GnRH analogues are often preferred for this indication.

Administration

Oestrogen is extensively metabolised in the liver (beware liver disease, clotting effects).

- orally, e.g. ethinyloestradiol 20 μg daily
- vaginally: creams, pessaries, impregnated ring pessary (very low doses possible)
- transdermally – patches or gel
- subcutaneous implant – 6 monthly approx.

Note: Natural oestrogens have a more favourable lipid profile and are preferred to synthetic formulations.

Important contraindications:

- oestrogen-dependent tumours
- liver disease
- thromboembolic history
- untreated hypertension

◆ Progestogens

Progesterone is produced by the corpus luteum and placenta and metabolised in the liver to pregnanediol. Progesterone assay is used to confirm ovulation. Progesterone has the following actions:

- pituitary inhibition of FSH and LH production
- raised body temperature (0.5°C)
- secretory changes (breast, uterus)
- decreased/viscous cervical mucus
- uterine contractions (slow)
- maintenance of pregnancy

Synthetic preparations are used therapeutically. They are classified into:

1. Natural derivatives – e.g. hydroxyprogesterone 250 mg i.m. twice weekly for early habitual abortions and long-acting medroxyprogesterone (Depo-Provera) 150 mg i.m. for contraception.

2. Testosterone derivatives – e.g. norethisterone (Primolut N) 5 mg t.d.s. used for dysfunctional uterine bleeding. It is metabolized to testosterone and is therefore not used to treat habitual abortion.
3. Stereo-isomers of progesterone – e.g. dydrogesterone (Duphaston) 10 mg b.d.
4. Newer, less androgenic, 'third generation' progestogens with more favourable arterial effects via better lipid profiles, e.g. desogestrel, gestodene, norgestimate, but adverse effects on thromboembolic risks.

Progesterones are also used in the combined pill, and high-dose progesterone (e.g. medroxyprogesterone 250 mg daily) is used to palliate advanced uterine carcinoma.

◆ Antiprogesterones

Useful antagonists have been developed to several of the five steroid hormones:

oestrogens	– clomiphene, tamoxifen
androgens	– cyproterone
progesterones	– mifepristone
mineralocorticoids	– spironolactone
glucocorticoids	

Antiprogesterones are being developed which are not androgenic and do not interfere with the synthesis of adrenal steroids. Progesterone is a key hormone in establishing and maintaining pregnancy. An antiprogesterone would therefore:
– induce menstruation (given in luteal phase)
– prevent implantation (given days 24–26)
– induce abortion (given in early pregnancy)

Antiprogesterones are now licensed for use in medical termination of pregnancy and prior to induction of labour following intrauterine death. Mifepristone (RU 486) is a progesterone receptor blocker causing detachment of the trophoblast, luteolysis and reduced HCG production. This leads to increased uterine contractility and also increases prostaglandin receptors (hence use in TOP).

◆ Primary amenorrhoea

Most girls have their first period before the age of 16. Other signs of puberty normally precede menstruation by about a year and if longer than 2 years then an absent uterus/vagina or an imperforate hymen is likely. No breast development by the age of 14 years merits investigation. There is a wide variation between normal girls in the timing of the stages of puberty:
– breast growth (8.5–13 years)
– pubic hair
– axillary hair
– growth spurt
– menarche

Primary amenorrhoea is best assessed according to whether these secondary sexual characteristics are present or absent (and whether they have developed according to their usual sequence) and by the presence or absence of signs of virilisation.

1. Secondary sexual characteristics present

– imperforate hymen
– absent vagina (XX) ± uterus
– absent vagina (XY – i.e. testicular feminisation)

If the vagina seems to be absent, perform a PR. A mass anteriorly suggests haematocolpos due to vaginal septum. If the vagina is absent, chromosomal analysis is necessary. If XX, renal ultrasound or IVU is important because renal anomalies are commonly associated.

An artificial vagina can be fashioned by forming an external perineal pouch (Williams' operation) which is enlarged initially with dilators. If ultrasound or laparoscopy reveals a normal uterus then an internal vagina can be constructed (McIndoe-Read operation). Referral to a surgeon specialising in adolescent gynaecology is appropriate.

2. Secondary sexual characteristics absent or poor

– constitutional
– hypothalamic (Kallman's syndrome: anosmia and specific failure to secrete FSH and LH)
– pituitary tumour
– ovarian dysgenesis (XO or XX)
– systemic or endocrine disease

Most cases are constitutional and there is usually a family history of late puberty in one parent to aid diagnosis.

If the girl is short (under 1.47 m – 4 foot 10 inches), Turner's syndrome (XO) must always be considered (poor height growth is due to overall loss of chromosomal material). In pure gonadal dysgenesis (XX) there are no sex hormones produced so the patient is tall (there is no or very late epiphyseal fusion) and FSH will be high.

After the age of 16 (or before if breast development, height or weight are delayed by more than 2 years), other causes must be excluded. Careful history and examination usually reveals any systemic ill-health (coeliac disease, thyroid dysfunction, renal tubular disease can be overlooked). Do not miss anorexia nervosa, now increasingly common in young girls tempted to diet by peer pressure. Serum thyroxine must always be estimated. Rare pituitary tumours (usually craniopharyngioma) may be excluded by cranial CT or X-ray, and gonadotrophin assays. Hyperprolactinaemia can rarely present with *primary* amenorrhoea.

3. Signs of virilisation

These include hirsutism, cliteromegaly, general muscular development. Consider:
– intersex (e.g. XY with cryptorchidism and hypogonadism)
– congenital adrenal hyperplasia (CAH)
– tumour (adrenal or ovarian)

Examine the genitalia for normality and the labia and groins for lumps (testes) and abdomen for large ovarian mass. Chromosomal analysis and hormone assays will be essential in every case and may lead to other tests (laparoscopy, adrenal scan).

Imperforate hymen

- breast and pubic hair normal
- cyclical (monthly) lower abdominal pain without bleeding
- urinary hesitancy and retention
- abdominal mass arising from the pelvis (haematocolpos)
- PR mass anteriorly
- bulging bluish membrane seen vaginally (often not seen until examined in theatre)

Ultrasound shows a fluid/mixed echo mass arising from the pelvis.

Treatment is by incision of the membrane under sterile conditions in theatre, followed by prescription of the combined oral contraceptive for 3–6 months to give the reassurance of a regular bleeding pattern while uterine size settles to normal. Subsequent fertility is not usually impaired.

Testicular feminisation

XY with normal testes but androgen insensitivity, hence the female phenotype develops, but female internal organs are absent due to Müllerian inhibitory factor. The appearances are of a normal girl, often attractive, with good breast development, but there is:

- no sexual hair
- short blind vagina
- absent uterus
- testes (intra-abdominal, inguinal, labial)
- high (i.e. male) testosterone level
- XY karyotype

Examination reveals an absent vagina and cervix. Diagnosis is by chromosomal analysis and serum testosterone. Orchidectomy is indicated because of the risk of malignant change in the gonads. Oestrogen replacement maintains breast development and prevents hot flushes. Careful counselling is always required: the patient is genetically male but will have been brought up female, and now also diagnosed infertile.

Also remember 5-α-reductase deficiency 46XY: peripheral insensitivity to testosterone so female appearance before puberty but male characteristics develop at puberty as testosterone levels rise. Presents to clinic as 'virilised' female. Nicknamed 'penis at twelve' by remote societies where it was first recognised.

Turner's syndrome

Ovarian dysgenesis (streak ovaries) with other abnormalities due to overall loss of chromosomal material (XO). A combination of short stature and absent secondary sexual characteristics is highly suggestive of Turner's syndrome. Adrenal androgens may allow sparse pubic and axillary hair development, confusing the diagnosis in young adolescents. Other features may or may not be present:

- webbed neck
- widely spaced nipples
- wide carrying-angle at elbow
- short metatarsals
- coarctation of the aorta or aortic stenosis
- peripheral oedema
- intelligence is usually normal

Turner's syndrome is diagnosed by chromosomal analysis (XO). It is treated in mid-teenage years (**Note**: maximise adult height before possible oestrogen effect on epiphyseal closure) with conjugated oestrogens (0.3 mg/day) for 3–6 months, increasing to 0.625–1.25 mg/day to achieve uterine and breast development. After 1 year, a progestogen should be added making a cyclical opposed regimen, e.g. conjugated oestrogens continuously + Provera 5 mg days 17–26; alternatively, synthetic ethinyloestradiol increasing from 5–50 μg/day with cyclical Provera. This causes breast development and cyclical bleeding and can be continued unchanged into adult life. It is replacement therapy and does not cause further stunting of growth.

Up to 10% of girls with Turner's syndrome may have some initial oestrogenisation, but fewer than 1/100 will have periods. There are reports of fertility, especially in mosaics. Raised gonadotrophin levels confirm eventual gonadal failure.

◆ Puberty

1. The *physical signs* of puberty are:
   - breast growth (average 11 years)
   - pubic hair
   - axillary hair
   - growth spurt
   - menstruation (average 13 years in UK)

   The changes occur due to hypothalamic maturation and also due to the synthesis (from adrenal precursors) of oestrogens in fat – the average *weight* at the menarche is 47 kg.

2. *Intersex* may first be recognised at puberty, either because of primary amenorrhoea due to testicular feminisation (XY) or a mild form of CAH (XX), or because the 'girl ' (in fact XY with cryptorchidism and hypospadias) develops cliteromegaly and a deep voice due to rising testosterone levels. Generally it is best to try to retain the sex to which the patient has adjusted psychologically.

3. Puberty may be *delayed* (see primary amenorrhoea).

4. *Precocious puberty* is defined as breast development before the age of 8 or periods before the age of 10. Pregnancy has been recorded at the age of 5.

   The possibilities are:
   - constitutional
   - hypothalamic tumour (CT scan) or postencephalitis
   - ovarian tumour (laparoscopy)
   - adrenal tumour (also virilised: raised oxo-steroids)

   Tumours must be excluded. Medroxyprogesterone or the anti-gonadotrophin, danazol can prevent menstruation and stunting of growth due to premature fusion of the epiphyses.

5. The *first cycles* are usually anovular, and heavy dysfunctional bleeding can occur. The girl and her mother can be reassured that it usually settles down after three or four cycles. (If it does not, ultrasound and EUA may be important to exclude an ovarian tumour.) Norethisterone 5 mg b.d. can be given for the week before the period and will reduce the loss. Iron-deficient anaemia

rarely develops in such a short space of time. A rare cause of excessive uterine bleeding in some countries is endometrial tuberculosis – diagnose by curettage for histology.

◆ Dysmenorrhoea

1. *Primary dysmenorrhoea* describes the colicky menstrual cramps that occur from day 1 of the period, with pain in the suprapubic region, low back and groins. The pain usually only occurs in ovulatory cycles, presumably because a raised progesterone is necessary to produce the high prostaglandin levels found in the menstrual fluid in these girls. Periods usually become painful soon after puberty once the cycles become ovulatory. Nausea, diarrhoea and flushing can occur. It is nearly always relieved after a vaginal birth – this may be partly due to relaxation at the cervical os. Reassurance and explanation are very important. There are three main approaches to treatment:
   a) analgesics and antispasmodics, e.g. hyoscine (Buscopan) 20 mg t.d.s.
   b) prostaglandin inhibitors, e.g. mefenamic acid (Ponstan) 500 mg q.d.s. Neurofen and other NSAIDs are also effective
   c) the combined pill to inhibit ovulation
   Cervical dilatation or presacral neurectomy are now very rarely used.
2. *Secondary* or *congestive dysmenorrhoea* occurs classically in older women with endometriosis or chronic salpingitis and may therefore be an indication for laparoscopy. The pain usually starts several days before the period, is constant rather than colicky and is often associated with back pain, deep dyspareunia and sometimes menorrhagia. The pelvic examination may show uterine fixity, enlargement or fibroids. When no pathology is found it is ascribed to pelvic congestion and the possibility of psychological/sexual problems should be considered.

◆ Premenstrual syndrome (PMS)

Definition: Cyclical recurrence in late luteal phase of a combination of distressing physical, psychological and/or behavioural changes of such severity as to cause deterioration in interpersonal relationships and/or interference with normal activity.

Symptoms disappear with onset of menstruation. Over 100 symptoms (50% physical, 50% behavioural) have been described – none is unique or diagnostic. The most common are:
- bloating, oedema, weight gain
- headaches
- breast swelling and pain
- change in bowel habit
- mood changes and irritability
- depression – sleep/sex/appetite/concentration affected

Standardised questionnaire devised by Moos (1968) remains the most widely used diagnostic tool (details >45 symptoms).

PMS is more common with increasing age, parity, longer intermenstrual intervals, family stresses and lack of exercise and relaxation.

Possible aetiological factors include excess oestrogen, progesterone deficiency, fluid retention, excess prolactin, B_6 deficiency, hypoglycaemia, prostaglandin excess or deficiency, hormone 'allergy', endogenous opiate effects and thyroid dysfunction, or may be purely psychogenic. The pathophysiology remains obscure!

Management

First, confirm the diagnosis, taking a comprehensive history (menstrual, social, sexual), then:
– reassure
– correct relevant causes
– relieve symptoms (empirical treatment usually)

All therapies work in some people; none is universally successful.
– progesterones in luteal phase (little evidence but no harm)
– lifestyle modification (diet and exercise)
– eliminate menstrual cycle (combined O/C, GnRH analogues, danazol, hysterectomy + BSO + HRT)
– pyridoxine 100 mg daily (avoid overdosage)

For particular symptoms treat the most severe first:
– mefenamic acid 500 mg t.d.s. (headache)
– spironolactone 100 mg daily, days 18–28 (fluid retention)
– dydrogesterone 10 mg b.d., days 12–26 (psychological symptoms)
– bromocriptine 5 mg nocte (mastalgia)

Dydrogesterone (Duphaston) has been shown to be more effective than placebo. In severe PMS, danazol 100–200 mg daily (continuously) is often effective where other measures have failed, and does not usually interfere with the menstrual pattern.

Most treatment is based on unsubstantiated theory. A conservative approach is therefore best, with support and reassurance (many women feel they are 'going mad'). Women may request hysterectomy – this can be useful if the periods themselves are debilitating after several days of severe PMS, but without oophorectomy cyclical (ovarian) symptoms will persist. More research is urgently needed.

◆ Heavy periods

Menorrhagia means heavy but regular periods. A menstrual calendar may be useful. Judge severity by:
– clots/flooding
– double protection (pads and towels)
– unable to work or go out
– iron-deficiency anaemia

May resolve spontaneously over time but consider *causes*:
– fibroids
– polyps (endometrial)
– adenomyosis
– IUD in situ?
– pelvic infection
– clotting disorder (rare)
– hypothyroidism

– dysfunctional uterine bleeding (no local pathology found, a diagnosis of exclusion after investigation)

Management
– exclude local cause, VE, remove IUD
– hysteroscopy and endometrial biopsy (outpatient procedure preferred to D&C) if aged over 40 years or other suggestive features
– check Hb and serum ferritin

If no cause found locally, try to establish management choice of the individual patient – medical *vs* surgical, prefers treatment *between* periods (hormonal) or *during* bleeding (non-hormonal). Consider future fertility and contraception. Choice depends on cycle pattern and length.

Medical
1. Non-hormonal: useful if cycle is predictable
   – mefenamic acid (Ponstan) 500 mg t.d.s. 2 days prior to and during bleeding
   – tranexamic acid (Cyclokapron) 1–1.5 g b.d. or q.d.s. during bleeding
   – ethamsylate (Dicynene) 500 mg q.d.s. during bleeding
2. Hormonal: necessary if cycle irregular
   – combined O/C (start with average (30 μg) dose oestrogen preparation, reducing later if possible)
   – norethisterone 5–10 mg b.d. days 10–26
   – medroxyprogesterone acetate 10 mg days 16–26
   – dydrogesterone 10 mg b.d. days 10–26
   – danazol 200–400 mg daily continously (especially good leading into menopause)
3. Combination of 1 and 2

Notes
– main side-effects in hormonal group – weight gain, bloating, breast tenderness
– use 3-month course, then review. Repeat second course if relapse
– use medroxyprogesterone acetate 15 mg stat then 5–15 mg/day to stop a prolonged bleed and refer for investigation

There are two basic types of dysfunctional bleeding:
a) ovulatory and regular – heavy bleeding is due to a poor luteal phase
b) anovular and chaotic. Typically the persistently high oestrogen levels cause 6–8 weeks amenorrhoea followed by heavy prolonged bleeding. The pattern is irregular and curettage is indicated to exclude pathology (incomplete abortion, polyp, carcinoma)

The traditional copper IUD is often linked to heavy periods. The woman may prefer to try a smaller copper device, change to the Mirena IUS (a progestogen-releasing IUD, see Chapter 3 *Family planning*) or use another method of contraception. Alternatively, antiprostaglandins can be used to decrease blood loss. Tranexamic acid is also effective (an antifibrinolytic which inhibits uterine fibrinolysins and decreases bleeding). It may cause nausea and is contraindicated when there is a history of thrombosis.

Surgical options for
treatment
– is hysterectomy and/or endometrial biopsy or D&C indicated?
– hysterectomy: abdominal/vaginal/laparoscopic? (ovarian conservation?)
– hysteroscopic surgery: options – transcervical resection of endometrium (TCRE)/laser ablation/radiofrequency ablation

Transcervical resection of endometrium
Increasingly common operation since mid-1980s. General or local anaesthetic and ideal day case procedure (cost-effective). Endometrium removed by loop diathermy approach via hysteroscopy and small submucous fibroids can also be removed easily. There is risk of uterine perforation at surgery. Histology of tissue removed is possible. Preoperative preparation with 6-week danazol or GnRH analogue therapy improves results as endometrium will be thinner (atrophic) at time of surgery. Also, postoperative depot injection improves results. Does not guarantee sterility and therefore often combined with laparoscopic sterilisation. Fluid loss into peritoneal cavity should be monitored to avoid postoperative overload.

Results better in expert hands but overall approx. 50% amenorrhoeic (mostly the women over 35), 35% lighter (tolerable) periods and 10–15% no change. These patients may go on to hysterectomy later. Overall 80% of the women in most studies are satisfied with the treatment. Long-term results (10 years or more) as yet unclear but, so far, no serious adverse events seem likely.

Laser ablation
Pioneered by Goldrath in USA, first reported in 1981 using Nd-YAG laser, hysteroscopy and D/Saline fluid distension medium. Subsequently Davis introduced technique in the UK, publishing in 1989. Heat conduction through the myometrium is minimal, tissue destruction is only a few mm. Low risk and can treat intrauterine adhesions also. Success rate similar to TCRE.

Radiofrequency ablation
Currently under investigation but shows promise. Differs from above methods as it does not offer direct visualisation of the procedure by hysteroscopy. There is no fluid distension medium and therefore no fluid overload problems. It takes around 20 minutes. The radiofrequency probe heats the endometrium. Higher amenorrhoea rate but risk of vesico-vaginal fistula if care not taken to shield the bladder (tissue penetration is greater than for laser methods).

This and other minimally invasive surgical techniques are the subject of RCOG surveys and are exciting developments in gynaecological surgery. Some randomised trials of hysteroscopic approaches *vs* hysterectomy suggest good outcomes for these techniques and fewer complications. Patient selection is probably important.

Bleeding disorders
Thrombocytopenia or Von Willebrand's disease can present (very rarely) with menorrhagia. If suspected (from bruising, bleeding or family history) measure platelet count/prothrombin time/KPTT. Von Willebrand's disease is dominantly inherited so there should be a family history. The above tests can all be normal and the diagnosis is

Managing period problems

NB: 'Dysfunctional uterine bleeding', by definition, means no pelvic or systemic pathology accounts for the symptoms. Its use should be reserved for women with no abnormalities on examination or investigation.

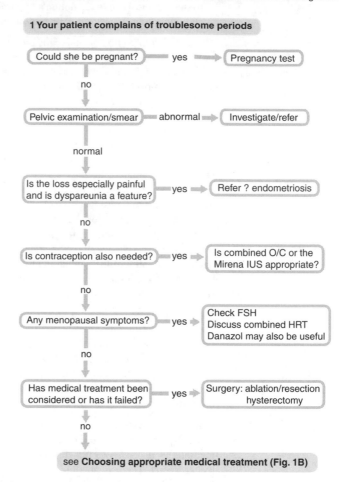

Fig. 1A Managing period problems

made on low Factor VIII levels (both coagulant and antigenic) and abnormal platelet aggregation (negative with ristocetin). Bleeding can be treated with fresh frozen plasma, but hysterectomy is usually necessary.

◆ Non-menstrual bleeding

- intermenstrual
- postcoital
- postmenopausal – suggests a carcinoma until proved otherwise
- breakthrough bleeding on O/C or depot methods
- abortion/ectopic pregnancy/trophoblastic disease

Managing period problems (Cont'd)

2 Choosing appropriate medical treatment

Treat logically, simple things first

Which group is your patient in?

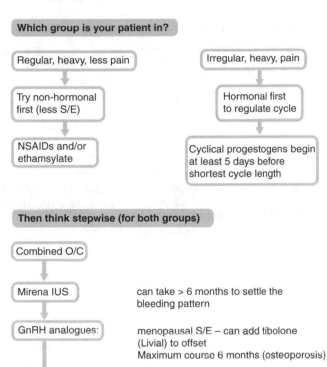

Fig. 1B Managing period problems

Consider also vaginitis, endometritis, cervical erosion/polyp.

Erratic bleeding in first 1–2 cycles of POP or combined O/C is common, as it is on HRT, and also after Mirena IUS insertion. Bleeding at an inappropriate time in cyclical HRT needs investigating, however.

Management

1. Always consider pregnancy. Check β-HCG.
2. Always consider carcinoma, especially in over-40s or in those with risk factors such as obesity, diabetes, unopposed oestrogen use.
3. Curettage or endometrial biopsy ('Pipelle' or 'Gynocheck') ± ovarian and endometrial thickness ultrasound usually indicated

(*always* for postmenopausal bleeding). Outpatient procedures are as reliable as formal D&C at picking up malignancy if hysteroscopy is available.

4. Laparoscopy may be indicated if erratic bleeding, positive HCG and no intrauterine pregnancy on ultrasound (for ectopic risk).

◆ Secondary amenorrhoea

Definition: the cessation of periods for more than 6 months.

Commonest causes are pregnancy and menopause. Otherwise 99% are due to endocrine causes and most respond readily to treatment except premature ovarian failure.

Consider:
- hypothalamic – weight loss, stress (45%)
                 – failure of feedback mechanisms (20%).
                     These respond to clomiphene
- hyperprolactinaemia (20%)
- premature ovarian failure (10%). Check FSH
- polycystic ovary syndrome (PCO) (4% – probably more in reality but diagnosis disputed)
- hypothyroidism (1%)

Rarely it may be due to hypopituitarism (Sheehan's syndrome after uterine haemorrhage), Cushing's syndrome, virilising tumours, Turner's mosaicism (XO/XX, when some periods can occur spontaneously), or uterine occlusion (Aschermann's syndrome after curettage or after TCRE).

Note: Post-pill amenorrhoea is usually indicative of a return to the pre-existing hormonal state before regular withdrawal bleeds occur on the O/C, and it responds to clomiphene in most cases.

Management

1. History
     – possibility of pregnancy (β-HCG)
     – weight loss, emotional upset
     – previous menstrual pattern
     – pill or other drugs
     – galactorrhoea
     – hot flushes
     – hirsutism (may be disguised)
     – general health (especially thyroid symptoms)

2. Examination
     – for hirsutism or signs of thyroid disorder
     – VE to exclude pregnancy and assess the size of the uterus/ovaries
     – ultrasound scan/serum HCG levels may be necessary to exclude pregnancy

3. Investigations. If the woman is obese and hirsute, she is usually assumed to have polycystic ovary syndrome (PCO). Check LH/FSH ratio. A serum testosterone is measured to exclude virilising tumours (when it would be extremely high). Clomiphene (may need 100 mg days 2–5 in PCO) will often induce ovulation.

The *progesterone challenge test* is useful (exclude pregnancy first). Norethisterone 5 mg b.d. or Provera 5 mg t.d.s. is given for 1 week: if a withdrawal bleed occurs then the woman must be well oestrogenised and is simply having anovular cycles. Both menstruation and fertility should return with clomiphene. This condition is said to be due to a 'cycle initiation defect' with a presumed inability of the hypothalamus to initiate normal follicular development that will proceed to ovulation. (In PCO oestrogen levels are high and progesterone would also cause a withdrawal bleed.) If progesterone fails to cause a withdrawal bleed then hormone assays are indicated:
- FSH (ovarian failure)
- prolactin
- free T4/TSH

4. If the cause is hypothalamic (normal hormone levels, no clinical features of PCO), it may be due to weight loss or stress. Losing more than 10 kg (unless the woman is already obese) tends to cause amenorrhoea and the woman need not necessarily have anorexia nervosa. Increased fitness and physical training will often cause menstrual cycle disturbance – probably due to change in the fat/muscle ratio – marathon runners, ballet dancers, etc. are often amenorrhoeic. Stresses such as travel, career change or family crisis may cause amenorrhoea. These problems may resolve and periods should return. Clomiphene is ineffective in these cases (because it cannot cause GnRH to rise) but injectable gonadotrophins/FSH (Metrodin) will induce ovulation if immediate fertility is required (but oestrogen levels need to be monitored). It is better to persuade the woman to regain weight, when periods and fertility should resume.

5. In premature ovarian failure (high FSH) natural fertility cannot be restored and only HRT or complex fertility treatment can be offered.

6. Temporary resistant ovary syndromes may occur (ovarian biopsy confirms germ cells present), but are rare.

7. Contraception is still necessary because the problem may resolve (weight loss, stress) or because sporadic ovulation may occur (PCO and cycle initiation defect). Patients with hypothalamic disorders are underoestrogenised and may require supplementation to offset the risk of osteoporosis (begin O/C or HRT). In PCO resting oestrogen levels are often high and these patients are at increased risk of endometrial hyperplasia. (Some authorities recommend inducing formal withdrawal bleeds to counter the effect on the endometrium – once or twice a year.) In hyperprolactinaemia the combined contraceptive pill was thought to cause enlargement of a pituitary tumour, but recent evidence suggests the pill is safe if taken with bromocriptine.

◆ Hyperprolactinaemia

High prolactin levels (above 4000 μU/ml) inhibit FSH and LH. The features are:
- amenorrhoea
- galactorrhoea (25%)
- pituitary tumour (40%)

A small tumour not demonstrated by tomography and CT scan is likely to be a microadenoma. Prolactin levels do not vary with the menstrual cycle but are elevated by stress, hence moderate elevation is common. The assay should always be repeated if the level is high. Drugs that are dopamine antagonists (phenothiazines, haloperidol, methyldopa, cimetidine, metoclopramide) will elevate prolactin, as will hypothyroidism. These must be excluded.

Treatment is with bromocriptine, a central dopamine agonist, which restores prolactin levels to normal almost immediately. Side-effects of nausea and postural hypotension are common so start with 2.5 mg after supper, gradually increasing to 5 mg t.d.s. If the woman gets pregnant on bromocriptine, visual fields must be monitored because a pituitary tumour can enlarge in pregnancy. If the tumour does start to enlarge, bromocriptine should be continued throughout the pregnancy.

If the pituitary tumour is of a significant size, the treatment of choice is a selective excision to avoid optic nerve compression, via a transphenoidal approach which does not cause later hypopituitarism. Microadenomas do not require surgical resection but should be closely monitored.

Galactorrhoea with normal periods cannot be due to hyperprolactinaemia and is usually due to repeated stimulation of the nipples, often sexual.

◆ Polycystic ovary syndrome (PCO)

Probable chain of events:
- obesity (increased conversion of androgens to oestrogen), hence
- low FSH
- high LH (possibly due to persistently high oestrogens), hence
- multiple lutein cysts, producing
- androstenedione (a 17-oxo-steroid), hence
- hirsutism, oligomenorrhoea or amenorrhoea

These patients are classically obese and hirsute but increasingly PCO is recognised in apparently normal women with oligomenorrhoea or amenorrhoea. Diagnosis is by history/examination:
- classical ultrasound appearance of ovaries: dense stroma, ring of small peripheral cysts
- increased LH/FSH ratio
- laparoscopic appearance of ovaries: smooth, enlarged, 'glossy'
- elevated plasma testosterone (but often normal range)

Management Weight loss in itself may improve the situation.

If fertility is required: clomiphene may induce ovulation (anti-oestrogen, increases endogenous production of FSH) but more direct ovarian stimulation by injections of pure FSH (Metrodin) then HCG, is often required. Risk of hyperstimulation with ovulation-induction regimens in PCO patients is greater than in non-PCO oligomenorrhoeic women. Prior down-regulation of LH levels by GnRH analogues improves the successful ovulation rate. Ovulation rates, however, are often not matched by conception rate.

If fertility is not required:
– contraception is still necessary (sporadic ovulation occurs)
– progesterone use (as in combined O/C) protects against endometrial hyperplasia if resting E2 levels are high
– symptomatic measures for hirsutism
– electrocautery of ovaries (laparoscopically) or wedge resection of ovaries has some benefits in resistant cases but is not widely used

◆ Hirsutism

Hirsutism is a common complaint and causes a lot of anxiety about both appearance and loss of femininity.

Males and females have the same number of hair follicles at birth. Hirsutism is due to sensitisation of male-pattern hair follicles by testosterone, possibly due to a temporary fall in sex hormone-binding globulin (SHBG) and a rise in free testosterone levels. Once activated, the hair continues to grow (hence hair growth tends to recur on stopping drug treatment).

A full history and examination is important. Ask about drugs (e.g. phenytoin, minoxidil, danazol or combined pills containing norgestrel), periods and family history. Examine to see full extent of hirsutism (most patients will already have self-treated – ask) and to exclude signs of virilisation (breast atrophy, cliteromegaly, unusual musculature). If hirsutism is mild and periods regular the woman may be reassured.

The following would indicate referral to a gynaecological endocrinologist, to exclude virilising tumours (which can be life-threatening):
– rapid progression of hair growth, hair growth in new sites (shoulders and back)
– reduced menses or infertility
– virilisation
– late-onset acne

Constitutional hirsutism

98% of cases are constitutional. The hirsutism is usually confined to the face and forearms and starts to develop from the time of puberty. There is usually a family history and it is particularly common in Southern European and Asian women. Periods are regular. Serum testosterone (a useful single screening test) is normal and can be a useful way of reassuring about femininity. Low SHBG levels usually predict a good response to oestrogens.

Treatment

Treatment is systemic and cosmetic.

Systemic treatment

First-line treatment is Dianette (ethinyloestradiol 35 µg, cyproterone acetate 2 mg). Oestrogens elevate SHBG and cyproterone is anti-androgen. It is particularly useful if there is also acne.
– other 35 µg oestrogen pills (to elevate SHBG levels)
– cyproterone acetate (anti-androgen)
– spironolactone (anti-androgen)
– dexamethasone 0.5 mg daily (suppression of androgens)

More severe cases of hirsutism may respond to higher doses of cyproterone, 50–100 mg daily, combined with 50 µg ethinyloestradiol for

17

menstrual regulation and contraception (Note: cyproterone can feminise a male fetus). Lethargy and breast tenderness sometimes occur but are usually mild. The initial course of treatment is 18–24 months. Improvement takes 3–6 months (the growth cycle of a hair follicle) and relapse is common.

Topical therapy Important because systemic therapy is long-term and hirsutism recurs when it is stopped. The mainstay of therapy is depilation. None of the depilatory methods increases hair growth. Methods include:
- shaving
- electrolysis (not available on the NHS)
- waxing
- depilatory creams
- plucking
- bleaching
- cosmetic make-up

Hirsutism due to raised androgen levels

Rarely, hirsutism is due to raised androgen levels. Periods become scanty. The possibilities are:
- polycystic ovary syndrome (PCO)
- virilising tumours (adrenal, ovarian)
- late presentation of congenital adrenal hyperplasia (CAH)
- Cushing's syndrome

PCO is suspected from the associated obesity and oligomenorrhoea. Ultrasound may be diagnostic, showing typical polycystic ovaries. The hirsutism may respond to the pill or can be treated with cyproterone acetate but this is highly teratogenic and the woman *must* also be on the pill. It takes 3–6 months to work (the growth cycle of the hair follicle).

Virilising tumours are suspected if hirsutism is prepubertal or suddenly develops some years after puberty. There are often other signs of virilisation (clitoral hypertrophy, breast atrophy, bitemporal balding and voice changes). Serum testosterone levels are very high. Cross-sectional imaging techniques (CT, MRI scans) and selective venous sampling from adrenal or ovarian veins may be diagnostic.

Mild CAH can present late and is diagnosed by raised urinary 17-oxo-steroids and raised plasma 17-hyroxyprogesterone (or its urinary metabolite pregnanetriol). Cortisone replacement is curative and hirsutism will regress slightly on treatment.

Cushing's syndrome is suspected from obesity, striae, glycosuria and hypertension. Diagnosis is confirmed by a raised midnight cortisol and failure to suppress cortisol level with low-dose dexamethasone (or, best of all, a raised 24-hour urinary free cortisol). The classic tests are:
1. High-dose dexamethasone test (a pituitary tumour will be suppressed).
2. ACTH assay (high if ectopic, e.g. oat cell carcinoma, low if adrenal tumour).
3. Urinary 17-oxo-steroids (high if adrenal carcinoma, low if adenoma).

◆ Infertility

The problem of infertility can largely be managed by the interested GP. About 10% of couples are involuntarily infertile. 1 in 6 of the population requires help at some time in their lives because of infertility. The average time taken for the normal couple to conceive is 6–8 cycles. 90% of fertile couples achieve pregnancy by 1 year and investigation is normally delayed until after 1 year of regular intercourse.

The causes are:
– coital factors
– defective ovulation (30%)
– defective sperm (30%)
– tubal blockage (20%)
– endometriosis (5%)
– hostile cervical mucus (5%)
– unexplained (15%)
– very rarely, chromosomal or uterine factors

Two or three factors may coexist. If the prognosis is hopeless, suitably sympathetic counselling and advice is needed – assisted conception with donor egg or sperm, AID, adoption.

Often the woman presents first, but the woman and her partner should be seen together whenever possible. It takes two to be infertile and male factors are involved in at least a third of cases.

Management A *possible* scheme of management is as follows:
1. Detailed history and examination of both partners. The problem should be taken seriously at the initial presentation. Differentiate between primary (*no* previous pregnancies, regardless of outcome) and secondary infertility. Make sure reported pregnancies were substantiated (could have been oligomenorrhoea). The couple will normally be hoping for referral, and delay in referral can be misconstrued as lack of interest. It is usually best to counsel about the optimum timing for intercourse (and pre-ovulation mucus changes) and to refer early to a specialist clinic. Self-testing kits detecting LH surge are sold in pharmacies but repeated use gets very expensive and adds little to the situation once ovulation and regular cycles have been confirmed. Ongoing advice, explanation and support are especially important for couples as they face a series of investigations and often long periods of waiting for the results of tests. For the 50% who fail to conceive the support of an interested GP is particularly important.
2. The GP should:
   – check for infected cervical ectropion and take a smear (if required)
   – swab cervix for chlamydia
   – screen for rubella antibodies and vaccinate before treatment if not immune
   – arrange semen analysis, including microbiological culture (collection technique important)
   – counsel/test for HIV if appropriate

19

A past history of STD, especially chlamydia, merits early referral to investigate for tubal disease. Semen analysis needs to be interpreted with caution unless there is obvious severe oligospermia (repeat if in doubt).

3. Always exclude pregnancy before beginning any treatment course (β-HCG – result same day). It is safe to treat with clomiphene 50 mg daily on days 2–6 of each cycle. Before treatment check:
   - prolactin (hyperprolactinaemia)
   - T4, TSH (hypothyroidism)
   - FSH/LH (premature menopause, PCO)
   - progesterone assay days 20–25 of cycle

   If pregnancy has not been achieved on clomiphene await specialist appointment. Send detailed letter plus all results. Clomiphene should only be given for 6 months.
   The following tests may be needed:
   - postcoital tests and/or ovulation detection of LH surge
   - progesterone assays
   - repeat hormone assays
   - laparoscopy and dye studies (checks tubal patency and inspects pelvis for adhesions/endometriosis/ovarian mobility)
   - HSG or USS using saline or contrast media ('Echovist') is sometimes appropriate and can delineate the internal shape of the uterus as well as tubal patency
   - endometrial histology with respect to cycle and dates (rarely TB or other uterine infections)

4. Liaise with specialists and maintain contact with couple for explanation and support. It is better to use the word 'subfertile' while the couple are still undergoing tests.

   If anovular cycles persist despite clomiphene 100 mg, arrange ultrasound to monitor follicular development/ovulation (in case of luteinised unruptured follicle syndrome). Specialist clinics are required to supervise use of GnRH and HCG because of the risk of hyperstimulation. Down-regulation with analogues before starting drugs such as Metrodin increases success. Frequent follicle and endometrial thickness assessment by ultrasound monitoring is mandatory. Hormonal assays can also be informative. Such precautions lessen the risk of ovarian hyperstimulation which can be life threatening, and reduce the chance of serious multiple pregnancies.

5. Use Fig. 2 to help in deciding which test is appropriate and when it is best performed.

Notes The couple should be seen together initially so they both clearly understand what will be involved. Ask about intercourse (technique and frequency) remembering that 'infertility' may be their way of presenting a psychosexual problem (vaginismus or impotence).

Ask the woman about her cycle (regularity, pain), dyspareunia, infections (postpartum or post-abortion) and gonorrhoea, and examine for fibroids or tenderness (endometriosis, infection).

Ask the man about his job (prolonged sitting can increase testicular temperature, e.g. driving), his general health (diet, exercise, smoking, alcohol), recent high fevers, drugs, previous infections and operations.

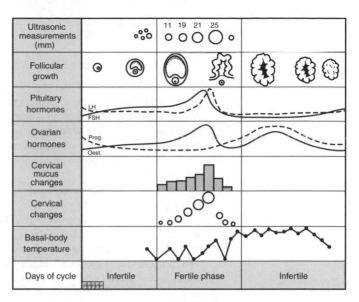

Fig. 2 Methods of measurements of fertility

Bilateral mumps, orchitis or late orchidopexy for undescended testis can cause oligospermia. Gonorrhoea or herniorrhaphy can damage and obstruct the vas deferens. TURP can cause retrograde ejaculation.

Examine standing for a varicocele, exclude hypospadias, assess testicular size, palpate the vas for thickening and perform a PR for tenderness (prostatitis). A simple hydrocele does not affect fertility.

Both the basal temperature charts and a special thermometer with 0.1°C readings can be prescribed. Explain that the oral temperature must be taken before rising each morning. Ovulation can occur 3 days either side of the rise in temperature. Temperature charting has been largely superseded by assay of serum progesterone, measured on day 21 of a 28 day cycle (when it should be above 30 mmol/l). If this is low, it confirms anovulation.

Clomiphene/tamoxifen/cyclofenil are anti-oestrogens that prevent oestrogen from inhibiting FSH – the FSH rise then initiates a normal cycle and ovulation.

If the woman has amenorrhoea, a progesterone-induced bleed will show that the endometrium is well oestrogenised: the amenorrhoea is probably due to anovular cycles and should respond to clomiphene. This challenge test confirms that the hypothalamic–pituitary–ovarian axis is substantially intact and suggests that anti-oestrogens should work.

The postcoital test (PCT) is the single most useful test in infertility. Cervical mucus is taken around day 14 of the cycle, the morning after intercourse, and should show at least 10 motile sperm per high power

field. Accurate timing is essential and the test needs special experience to interpret properly. If the count is normal it proves that:
- coitus is effective
- cervical mucus is adequate (implying ovulation)
- sperm is normal

If poor, check timing, repeat history, examination and semen analysis with culture. If non-motile, and smear/swabs show infection, repeat the test after a course of antibiotics; otherwise, ovulation stimulation may help to improve the quality of cervical mucus (except clomiphene which can have a marked anti-oestrogenic effect on mucus in some women).

Repeat the postcoital test. If still non-motile, consider a sperm–mucus penetration test (in vitro). Sperm penetration of pre-ovulatory cervical mucus is twice as good as seminal analysis at predicting fertility. If the PCT is poor and semen analysis is normal, sperm–mucus penetration tests may show sperm clumping and poor penetration (look for anti-sperm antibodies in the man's serum) or sperm immobilisation by mucus (look for antibodies in the woman's serum). Anti-sperm antibody levels can be checked although these are not helpful for prognosis. Intrauterine insemination of fresh semen at the time of ovulation can be tried (IUI). Assisted conception offers new hope to these couples.

◆ Male infertility

If the sperm count is poor, seminal analysis should always be repeated because there is daily fluctuation, and viral illness or fever can cause a low count for 3 months. A masturbation specimen is collected after 3 days' abstinence directly into a sterile plastic container, kept at room temperature and then examined by an experienced seminologist within 2 hours.

There should be *at least*:
- 2 ml
- 20 million/ml
- 75% motile
- 75% normal morphology

A *low count* may be due to:
- varicocele (examine standing)
- raised testicular temperature
- prostatitis
- drugs (alcohol, cyclophosphamide, nitrofurantoin)
- heavy smoking
- testicular atrophy (trauma, infection, hypopituitarism, XXY)

In unexplained infertility where semen analysis is normal, laboratory examination of sperm–egg interactions (as in IVF) can be both a treatment and provide clues as to the diagnosis. Male infertility is complex and early referral (preferably to an IVF unit) is recommended.

Management
1. Advise reduction of smoking or excessive alcohol consumption. If a varicocele is present, bilateral supra-inguinal ligation of the spermatic veins can restore fertility in up to 70%. If the testes are small and there is gynaecomastia, exclude Klinefelter's syndrome (XXY) by chromosomal analysis.
2. Advise cold scrotal douches, avoidance of long hot baths, boxer shorts and regular exercise, and repeat the seminal analysis in 3 months (each complete cycle of sperm production takes 3 months).
3. If prostatitis is suspected (tenderness PR, culture results), a 3-month course of rotating antibiotics (e.g. septrin, erythromycin, tetracycline) can sometimes improve the count.
4. If the count remains low then tamoxifen or clomiphene (to increase FSH), or mesterolone 100 mg daily, can be tried. (Testosterone inhibits FSH and actually *lowers* the count.) There is no evidence, however, that these empirical treatments help. Low counts are not a complete bar to fertility and it is best to maintain some hope for the couple while pursuing appropriate tests and referrals. Refer to an assisted conception unit.
5. Note that hormone assays and testicular biopsy are not routinely necessary. Pituitary failure will be suspected clinically (tiredness, impotence, pale hairless skin). Degeneration of the seminiferous tubules will be suspected from small testes but biopsy does not alter management.
6. If there is total aspermia, then FSH and testicular biopsy become useful tests to distinguish blocked ducts (normal testes, normal FSH) from testicular failure (small testes, high FSH, irreversible).
   In obstruction, a vasogram can be performed to exclude non-surgical obstruction deep at the ejaculatory ducts and epididymovasotomy may be performed (but results are still poor). If no block is demonstrated, testicular biopsy may show spermatogenic arrest (normal FSH) which may respond to gonadotrophins.
   Note: FSH stimulates *sperm production*
   LH stimulates *testosterone secretion*
7. If the sperm count is normal, the male may still be responsible for infertility due to IgG anti-sperm antibodies (suspected by clumping of sperm on a postcoital test and the MAR test). It is difficult to treat, but prescribing a short course of steroids the week before the woman's period can be tried. Antibody levels may fall but pregnancy rates often remain unchanged. Considerable risk and side-effects exist as the dose is high.
8. Infertility due to cervical hostility, hypospadias or poor sperm volume may be overcome by AIH/IUI with washed sperm.

◆ Assisted conception techniques

Advances in this field occur very rapidly. DRCOG candidates should know the basics: the main options are in-vitro fertilisation (IVF), gamete intrafallopian transfer (GIFT), intracytoplasmic sperm injection (ICSI) and intrauterine insemination (IUI). There are many developments (with appropriate acronyms!) and variants of all the techniques may be appropriate in certain cases. These treatments are rarely available on the NHS. The 'take-home' baby rate for GIFT and IVF is about 20%. There is no evidence that IVF increases the chance of fetal abnormality.

IVF and its associated procedures may also permit pre-implantation diagnosis by analysis of individual cells in the blastocyst, or by genetic analysis of the egg/sperm DNA and are therefore sometimes appropriate for couples without infertility but who carry rare genetic disorders.

These treatments are regulated by the Human Fertilisation and Embryology Authority (HFE Act, 1990) which licenses, inspects and governs treatment centres.

Indications
- tubal occlusion
- male infertility: oligospermia, antibodies (probably the most favourable for succesful treatment in male-factor infertility)
- ovulatory problems: oocyte not released at ovulation, drugs assisting ovulation but not producing viable in-utero pregnancies, early miscarriages
- pelvic endometriosis
- unexplained infertility
- pre-implantation diagnosis

Most centres now use controlled cycles (rather than spontaneous), giving optimal timing of treatment procedures.

IVF
The procedure involves:
- initial visit, assessment/screening, counselling and planning
- down-regulation
- follicle stimulation using clomiphene/GnRH. This increases the multiple pregnancy rate (15%) but transferring 3 embryos increases the success rate considerably. Subsequent embryo reduction may be offered for high multiples (5 or 6) and is legal
- monitoring: serial scans for follicular development and endometrial response (thickness and reflectivity) ± serial hormone levels
- timed HCG injection to mimic LH surge: pre-ovulatory follicles are harvested by laparoscopy or USS-guided needle aspiration. Eggs are checked by an embryologist and then incubated with fresh prepared semen
- the best fertilised embryos are later transferred (transcervically)
- follow-up: HCG testing and USS
- luteal and early pregnancy hormonal support

Success rate: reports vary from 10% to 30% but higher in selected cases. Highest rate for pure tubal damage, lowest for male factors. Success rate falls dramatically for older women and after multiple unsuccessful attempts.

GIFT
Originally popular as a DGH procedure (cheaper as no embryologist/culture facilities required) but best results are obtained if provided by centres with additional IVF resources. This is partly because in unexplained infertility, using GIFT alone does not offer insight into the cause of sperm–egg interaction failure (IVF in a lab setting does).

- follicle stimulation, sperm preparation and egg collection as above
- sperm and eggs are mixed in a small amount of culture medium, introduced into the fimbrial end of one or both tubes (same laparoscopy as used for egg collection)
- fertilisation is presumed to occur in the tube and implantation follows naturally. The technique is unsuitable for damaged tubes and does not allow for lab confirmation of satisfactory fertilisation

ICSI Capacitation and acrosome reaction in the sperm are not necessary for fertilisation as sperm are injected directly into the oocyte. Suitable for immature sperm or poor quality/small numbers. Sperm can be harvested from epididymis or testis thus ICSI can revolutionise the outlook for male infertility problems.

Developments
- better understanding of egg–sperm interaction
- pre-transfer study of the embryo offers the chance to make additional prenatal diagnosis of genetic defects
- donor eggs or sperm may be used (eggs from donors at sterilisation procedures)
- cryopreservation allows spare embryos to be stored or used for research (time limit imposed). New legislation now permits freezing of *eggs*. Previously, only semen and embryos could be frozen. Egg donors must be under 35 years
- cloning (already succesful in animal species)

The ethical issues of assisted conception

These continue to be debated widely. The Warnock Report (1984) was the Government's initial response to public concern over the social, ethical and legal issues of IVF in terms of both the treatment of infertility and research on human embryos.

The main recommendations were:
1. A new statutory *licensing authority* to regulate both infertility services and research projects.
2. IVF clinics (and AID clinics) should be licensed.
3. Services for IVF should be expanded within the NHS.
4. Agencies (commercial or otherwise) recruiting women for *surrogate pregnancies* ('womb-leasing') should be illegal (but individuals entering into private surrogacy arrangements will not be liable to criminal prosecution).
5. Children born by IVF or AID should not be branded as illegitimate (changes in legislation were recommended and later introduced).
6. *Egg donation* should be accepted and subject to the same controls as AID.
7. *Embryo donation* should be accepted provided that the semen and egg are brought together in vitro.
8. *Spare embryos* may be frozen and stored for repeated attempts. The right to use or dispose of the embryos should pass to the storage authority after 10 years (or in the event of the death of both parents).
9. *Research on embryos* should be legal up to 14 days (when the primitive streak appears) and it should be legal to create embryos

solely for experimentation (e.g. by rescuing ova from women undergoing sterilisation and fertilising them from a donor bank).

Embryo research Some people are opposed to embryo research, taking the view that a human being is created at the moment of fertilisation. Most people, however, accept that an embryo does not command the rights and privileges of a fully formed person, and that research on human embryos will bring important advances for the benefit of the community. Allowing research up to 14 days is a compromise between these two views, although many feel that 6 weeks would be a more realistic limit.

Embryo research may yield important new information on cell interaction, cell differentiation, tissue organisation and the causation and methods of prevention of congenital malformations. It may become possible to diagnose genetic disorders in the blastocyst prior to implantation (avoiding the need for late termination) and gene insertion techniques may one day cure diseases caused by defective genes.

Current research is concentrating on ways of improving assisted conception techniques and the success rate rises every year. Individual centres are researching a new contraceptive pill, male infertility and genetic abnormalities in the pre-embryo (the term for the fertilised ovum up to day 14).

Risks of assisted conception techniques
- ovarian hyperstimulation syndrome (cysts, ascites, pain, electrolyte imbalance – can be fatal)
- hazards of collection/replacement method (pain, infection, haemorrhage)
- ectopic more common
- multiple pregnancy and sequelae

◆ Spontaneous miscarriage

Note: the term *miscarriage* is preferred over the less sensitive *abortion* in front of patients.

Classification
- threatened
- inevitable
- complete
- incomplete
- septic
- recurrent
- missed

Presentation
- bleeding in early pregnancy (< 24 weeks)
- positive pregnancy test (or β-HCG) at some stage
- may have passed products
- pain is a frequent symptom

Ask about:
- length of amenorrhoea
- previous cycle/contraception
- positive test yet?
- symptoms of pregnancy?
- pain? (ectopic?)

Examination
- signs of pregnancy
- maternal condition – ?shocked
- amount of bleeding
- products seen?
- uterine size (? = gestation or not)
- os open or closed?
- adnexal mass or tenderness

Management
- resuscitation
- β-HCG if pregnancy not yet confirmed
- check viability with ultrasound if os closed or uterine size/dates discrepancy (positive fetal heart after 10-weeks gestation is associated with 95% success in maintaining pregnancy to term)
- take blood for Hb and group/save
- anti D if Rhesus negative (now not recommended unless > 12 weeks)
- NBM if waiting for theatre and ERPC

Note: Products stuck in os produce shock which exceeds degree of haemorrhage, due to vagal stimulation – check with speculum and remove if present.

If bleeding is heavy, ergometrine 0.5 mg i.m. (can be given i.v. by a doctor). Syntocinon infusion (40 U in 500 ml N saline) is useful while awaiting transfer to theatre.

Threatened miscarriage
- usually painless bleeding
- uterine size = dates
- os closed
- 75% settle spontaneously
- anti D is still required if over 12 weeks
- bed rest of unproven value but frequently advised
- USS confirms gestation (and intrauterine implantation)
- serum HCG continues to rise appropriately

Septic miscarriage
Fever, offensive discharge, tender.
- take HVS, blood cultures
- broad-spectrum antibiotics *prior* to evacuation
- risk of tubal damage if infection severe

Recurrent or habitual miscarriage
Defined as three or more *consecutive* miscarriages.

Causes:
- chronic maternal conditions: chronic renal disease, thrombophilia, Factor V Leiden mutation, antiphospholipid syndrome, SLE. Possibly diabetes and thyroid disease – but more often these women are subfertile and *not* miscarrying repeatedly
- immunological or unknown (50%)
- cervical incompetence (if second trimester losses)
- abnormal uterus (bicornuate/septate), fibroids
- parental chromosomes, especially translocations
- cytotoxic drugs/radiotherapy

Take a *careful* history to distinguish oligomenorrhoea with heavy menses from genuine pregnancy losses (positive test, products seen?, histology?).

Classical cervical incompetence causes sudden mid-trimester losses with few contractions. Check for previous TOP or cone biopsy. Diagnosis is by USS or HSG (hysterosalpinography) (cervical canal > 10 mm diameter). VE at booking is rarely diagnostic but may influence decision to insert a cervical suture. Vaginal insertion (under general anaesthetic) of a nylon (or inert tape) cervical suture at 14–16 weeks gestation is effective but should be reserved for genuine cervical incompetence cases as there is a significant risk of sepsis and/or preterm labour. The suture is removed vaginally (no anaesthetic required) at 37–38 weeks or at elective caesarean delivery. Most will require sutures in all subsequent pregnancies. Transabdominal cervical cerclage is appropriate in certain circumstances.

50% of first trimester losses appear to involve a chromosomal anomaly, usually sporadic, in the fetus. Importantly, even after three consecutive miscarriages the chance of success in the fourth is around 75% with no treatment, so the true value of the many suggested therapies is hard to assess.

Several bodies of research have suggested a failure of maternal immunoglobulin 'blocking' systems, causing rejection of the fetus. These women also have a higher incidence of pre-eclampsia, possibly also an immunological condition. Immunisation of the woman with her partner's lymphocytes or with antigens derived from trophoblastic tissue was popular (and produces pregnancy successes in about 75% of couples) but the evidence for definite therapeutic benefit is weak and immune and other disorders subsequently affected treated women.

Chromosomal abnormalities in the fetus are less common in habitual miscarriage than in sporadic cases. 4% of couples have chromosomal anomalies although often not the same as those in the fetus. Parents with chromosome translocations have a particularly high risk of further abnormal pregnancies and genetic counselling is advisable.

Treatment   Treat any underlying medical cause. For thrombophilias, low-dose aspirin (75 mg daily) has been found to be beneficial. These women are at greater risk of thromboembolic complications of pregnancy (heparin prophylaxis), IUGR and late fetal loss: specialist advice should be sought.

Various other therapies have been tried for early pregnancy loss but none shows any strong evidence of success. Options include HCG injections, depot progestogens and folate. Hormonal support in early pregnancy does seem important after IVF pregnancy.

Recurrent miscarriage clinics can offer advice and support and report greater success than general gynaecology clinics. Regular USS and positive reinforcement seem to have therapeutic (psychological?) benefits.

◆ Therapeutic abortion

Relevant legal events:
1929 Infant Life Preservation Act
1967 Abortion Act
1990 Human Fertilisation and Embryology Act

The Abortion Act requires two doctors to certify (on Form A, the 'blue form') that they have seen and/or examined the patient and are of the opinion that one of the following *clauses* applies:

a) The continuance of the pregnancy would involve risk to the life of the pregnant woman greater than if the pregnancy were terminated.
b) The termination is necessary to prevent grave permanent injury to the physical or mental health of the pregnant woman.
c) The pregnancy has NOT exceeded its 24th week and the continuance of the pregnancy would involve risk, greater than if the pregnancy were terminated, of injury to the physical and mental health of the pregnant woman.
d) The pregnancy has NOT exceeded its 24th week and the continuance of the pregnancy would involve risk, greater than if the pregnancy were terminated, of injury to the physical or mental health of any existing child(ren) of the family of the pregnant woman.
e) There is a substantial risk that if the child were born it would suffer from some physical or mental abnormalities as to be seriously handicapped.

Clause c) is the one used for most 'social requests' for TOP. At more advanced gestations TOP needs to be discussed extremely carefully, especially if there is a risk of the fetus being born alive (defined as being with any signs of life, even just a heartbeat). Note that for Clause e) TOP is legally allowed at any gestation, although moral and ethical considerations may argue against very late TOP for non-lethal abnormalities such as trisomy 21.

Form C (yellow) is completed later as notification by the doctor performing the TOP (statistics are collected annually). There are around over 150 000 legal terminations annually in England and Wales, at least 30% performed outside the NHS.

Any doctor, nurse or midwife may opt not to participate in TOP.

Safety and complications

In the first trimester TOP is a safe procedure (mortality 1/million esti mated pregnancies). In the 1994–96 Maternal Mortality Report there was 1 death from legal abortion and 2 from spontaneous miscarriage. First trimester termination is less likely to cause morbidity or mortality than continuing the pregnancy. Complications rise steeply with advancing gestation.

Immediate complications

– maternal mortality: shock, surgical, anaesthetic
– uterine damage: perforation, cervical tears or laceration
– haemorrhage
– incomplete procedure: retained products, sepsis

– failed termination: under 6 weeks gestation surgical TOP risks missing the gestation sac; medical TOP is preferable <7weeks
– infection (take swabs when TOP arranged)

Post-abortion sepsis is reduced by 50% using routine prophylaxis for chlamydia, gonococcus and bacterial vaginosis, with metronidazole 1 g p.r. at procedure + doxycycline 100 mg b.d. for 7 days afterwards.

Long-term sequelae
– psychiatric morbidity (counselling services important but often not well provided in hospital setting)
– infertility: dependent largely on infection
– ectopic pregnancy (secondary to tubal damage with infection)
– cervical incompetence/preterm labour (rare after first trimester procedures)

Methods
1. *<9 weeks (63 completed days).* Medical TOP: Mifepristone 200 mg orally followed after 36–48 hours by p.v. prostaglandin pessary, an E1 analogue (gemeprost, which is expensive, or misoprostol, which is much cheaper, and as effective before 7 weeks) is effective in 98% of cases before 7 weeks, and in 95% of cases between 7 and 9 weeks. Misoprostol can be used orally but vaginal administration is better for cervical ripening and TOP although administration by the vaginal route is unlicensed in the UK at the moment. Abortion is usually complete 6–8 hours after the prostaglandin (a small minority require ERPC). Need accurate dating by USS, and ideally do USS after procedure to check that it has been complete.
2. *<12–14 weeks.* Suction or vacuum aspiration. In England and Wales, general anaesthetic is usual but the procedure is frequently done under local elsewhere.
3. *>14 weeks.*
   – dilatation and evacuation (more popular in specialist private sector than in NHS)
   – prostaglandin: several routes – oral mifepristone followed by repeated prostaglandin (misoprostol or gemeprost) pessaries p.v. is commonest but intra-amniotic or extra-amniotic routes may be used. Epidural or opiate analgesia is often required. ERPC is often required before 24 weeks. Feticide should be considered if over 20 weeks, e.g. for fetal abnormality (by intracardiac injection of KCl under USS control)
   – other hypertonic solutions (saline/urea) have been used by intra-amniotic injection but there are other risks
   – hysterotomy. Rarely used nowadays but is indicated where uterine contractions carry a significant risk of uterine rupture due to previous uterine surgery. The scar is in the upper segment and itself carries a significant risk of rupture in a subsequent pregnancy

Notes
1. *Contraception should begin immediately after the TOP.* Ovulation occurs in the first cycle following TOP in over 90% of women.
2. *Selected feticide in an ongoing pregnancy*: in special circumstances one or more fetuses of a multiple pregnancy may legally be terminated whilst allowing the remaining ones to proceed.

The procedure usually involves selective transamniotic intracardiac injection of K^+ or air, killing that fetus. It can be used in high-order multiple pregnancies after IVF (e.g. reducing sextuplets to twins or triplets) or if one fetus is known to be congenitally abnormal. (**Note**: check no anastomotic vascular connections between fetuses, e.g. shared placenta vessels.)

3. *Counselling* is vitally important. Arrange genetic testing of fetus/parents and genetics opinion if required. Encourage post-mortem if TOP for fetal abnormality. Disposal and burial arrangements are allowed in the UK following fetal abnormality TOP or spontaneous loss > 14 weeks. Support groups exist, e.g. ARC (Antenatal Results and Choices).

◆ Tubal pregnancy

Roughly 0.5–1% of pregnancies in the UK are ectopic and almost all of these are tubal. Usually the cause is unknown but there may be a history of:
- tubal surgery, including infertility procedures or sterilisation
- IUD or POP (see family planning chapter)
- pelvic sepsis – accounts for 30%, especially chlamydia or gonorrhoea
- pelvic tuberculosis in relevant areas of the world
- assisted conception pregnancies (GIFT or IVF)

The site of the ectopic may affect the presentation. Common *symptoms* are:
- a missed period (may have had pregnancy test)
- dizziness or fainting
- pelvic or abdominal pain that usually precedes any vaginal bleeding. Can be over several weeks. Rarely, peritonism presents acutely with shoulder tip pain or upper abdominal pain
- vaginal bleeding which can be heavy

90% of tubal ectopics are ampullary, occurring in the free end of the fallopian tube, and rupture or abortion occurs at 6–9 weeks' gestation. Abdominal pain can be colicky (tubal peristalsis) or continuous, sometimes with peritonism (due to bleeding from the tube).

Vaginal bleeding can be slight and dark, coming from the endometrial decidua no longer supported by HCG, or it can be fresh red bleeding coming down the tube from ruptured vessels. The amount is not indicative of the diagnosis.

VE shows marked cervical excitation due to pelvic irritation. The uterus may feel bulky, and sometimes a tender mass is felt in one fornix (usually only able to feel this before rupture as it is too tender after), or a large posterior mass due to haematoma.

Differential diagnosis:
- threatened abortion (bleeding often before, or without, pain)
- salpingitis (fever, bilateral tenderness, short history of hours/days)
- appendicitis (fever, thirsty, ketotic, nausea, diarrhoea)
- ovarian cyst: torsion or rupture (severe pain, no bleeding)

Investigations
1. Simple *urinary HCG*: positive in > 95%.
2. *Ultrasound.* Ectopic and intrauterine pregnancies coexist in only 1 in 30 000 (more in IVF) so an intrauterine pregnancy (fetal pole seen) on scan almost excludes the diagnosis although a bright endometrium and pseudosac may be seen in association with ectopics. *Transvaginal USS* is especially accurate as definition of the adnexal region is so good, an early fetal pole can be measured (and dated) and pelvic free fluid is easily seen.
3. *Serial serum HCG levels* should be taken (0 and 48 hrs) if the diagnosis is unclear and ongoing intrauterine gestation is too early to be confirmed on vaginal USS. This will distinguish between complete abortion, 'blighted ovum' (USS = sac only), resolving tubal abortion or ongoing early pregnancy (which might be intra- or extrauterine), and may allow conservative management rather than immediate recourse to laparoscopy.
4. *Laparoscopy.* Perform if serum β-HCG significantly elevated (> 1000 IU) or rising on repeat test with no intrauterine pregnancy on USS. Most ectopic surgery is now performed to conserve the tube by linear salpingotomy, expressing the sac and conserving the tube. Laparoscopic surgery has revolutionised the hospital care of ectopic pregnancy and > 85% of cases are suitable. Laparotomy is usually only needed if haemorrhage is extensive, e.g. cornual pregnancy, or if the surgeon is too inexperienced to perform laparoscopic surgery safely. It is important to avoid simultaneous tubal surgery to the other tube, however tempting.

Notes
Diagnosis is notoriously difficult, and tubal pregnancy can be painless and present merely as a late 'period'. 10% occur in the interstitial part of the tube (isthmus or cornua) and tend to rupture early with massive intraperitoneal haemorrhage. The woman's period may only be a few days late when she develops severe abdominal pain, shock and generalised abdominal tenderness and rebound with slight distension. There may be no vaginal bleeding. Fig. 3 illustrates a management scheme suitable for a premenopausal patient presenting with acute pelvic pain.

Ectopic pregnancy remains an important cause of maternal mortality: 12 deaths (= 0.4/1000 ectopic pregnancies) in the 1994–96 Maternal Mortality Report. Two of these deaths from ectopic were judged to have followed such sudden and severe collapse that effective medical intervention was impossible. The key points are to make a prompt diagnosis where possible, resuscitate and operate immediately.

◆ Bartholin's cyst

Anatomy: a single Bartholin's gland lies approximately 0.5 cm deep to the posterior end of the labia minora on each side. The duct opens just inside the introitus, below the hymen. Normally the gland is not palpable.
– Bartholin's cyst: painless swelling, posterior 1/3, due to duct obstruction and retention of secretions. Can be recurrent
– Bartholin's abscess: painful, red, tender, sometimes fluctuant

Acute pelvic pain (in a premenopausal patient)

* Unknown patient in collapse state: assume ectopic, resuscitate in theatre asap
*Deterioration in clinical condition during investigation: laparoscopy ? ectopic

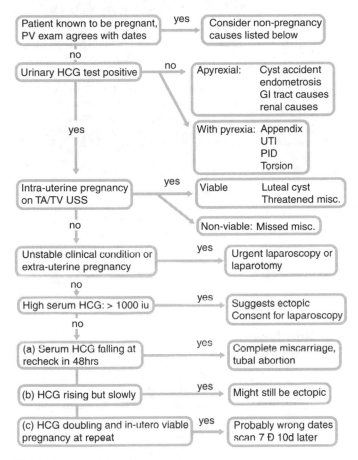

Patient complains of sudden onset of pelvic pain

Patient known to be pregnant, PV exam agrees with dates — yes → Consider non-pregnancy causes listed below

no

Urinary HCG test positive — no → Apyrexial: Cyst accident / endometrosis / GI tract causes / renal causes

With pyrexia: Appendix / UTI / PID / Torsion

yes

Intra-uterine pregnancy on TA/TV USS — yes → Viable: Luteal cyst / Threatened misc.

Non-viable: Missed misc.

no

Unstable clinical condition or extra-uterine pregnancy — yes → Urgent laparoscopy or laparotomy

no

High serum HCG: > 1000 iu — yes → Suggests ectopic / Consent for laparoscopy

no

(a) Serum HCG falling at recheck in 48hrs — yes → Complete miscarriage, tubal abortion

(b) HCG rising but slowly — yes → Might still be ectopic

(c) HCG doubling and in-utero viable pregnancy at repeat — yes → Probably wrong dates scan 7 Ð 10d later

Fig. 3 Acute pelvic pain

Treatment: best by marsupialisation for both cyst and abscess. De-roof the cyst, drain cavity, suture cyst wall to skin to allow continued drainage. Early antibiotic treatment is of little value, although antibiotics speed healing after abscess drainage. Excising the gland surgically is difficult and often incomplete.

◆ Pruritus vulvae

Associations:
- vaginal discharge (check for foreign body)
- infection (candida, warts)
- incontinence
- skin disorder (eczema, psoriasis, generalised pruritus)
- contact sensitivity
- vulval dystrophy: refer for diagnostic biopsy
- infestation (threadworms, scabies, lice)
- psychogenic

Diagnosis can be difficult because scratching causes secondary hypertrophic changes. Ask about vaginal discharge, inspect carefully, take a smear and swab if necessary and remember threadworms (especially in children). *Always exclude glycosuria.*

Treat any infection, remembering to treat the partner if necessary. Stop all applications. Contact sensitivity (to deodorants, spermicides, antiseptics) can be proved by patch testing.

If no cause is found, treat with a 1–2 week course of mild topical steroid (e.g. 1% hydrocortisone) and an oral antihistamine at night, e.g. promethazine (Phenergan) 50 mg, which is also a sedative and has a 12-hour action.

Recommend regular washing (avoiding soaps, although babycare products are usually OK) as perianal microorganisms contaminate the vulva, particularly in the elderly and in children, careful drying (a hair dryer is useful) and avoidance of tight nylon underwear or nightwear (warmth and moisture cause maceration).

Pruritus vulvae is not infrequently a symptom which points to underlying psychological problems, which may be of a psychosexual nature.

◆ Vulvodynia

Means chronic vulval dicomfort – often described as burning pain, stinging etc., particularly on pressure. Many suggested causes including viral/chronic infection but the answer is rarely found in any one individual. Includes dermatoses (lichen planus, lichen sclerosis and eczema), vestibulitis (candida implicated) and cyclical vulvodynia (symptoms recur in association with menses or coitus).

Management is symptomatic relief:
- simple analgesia is usually ineffective
- low-dose tricyclics (amitriptyline 25 mg nocte) are best
- emollient creams for eczema
- topical corticosteroid (Trimovate) is useful

Note: Colposcopic examination of the vulva can highlight areas appropriate for biopsy.

◆ Disorders of the vulval epithelium

The term 'vulval dystrophy' is not no longer appropriate: divide the problem into neoplastic and non-neoplastic.

Vulval intraepithelial neoplasia (VIN)

Often asymptomatic but can present with pigmentation, ulceration or hyperkeratotic (white) lesions. Pruritus is common (>50%).

Usually multifocal, diagnosed by vulval biopsy. Colposcopic inspection reveals mosaicism and permits directed biopsies. Graded I, II or III in similar way to CIN. VIN III may progress to invasive disease.

Treat by laser, simple vulvectomy or excision. Recurrence tends to occur because of the multifocal nature of the condition.

Paget's disease is a non-squamous condition, sometimes (25%) seen in association with adenocarcinoma elsewhere. Treat by wide local excision. It can resemble eczematous lesions – biopsy if in doubt.

Non-neoplastic epithelial conditions

– 'Lichen sclerosus': usually atrophic, thin and dry (labial adhesions common) but can be thickened, fissured and bleeding. The hyperkeratotic type is associated with squamous carcinoma of the vulva – biopsy and follow yearly. Symptomatic relief (pruritus and scratching) with hydrocortisone 1% ointment ± antihistamine orally (be careful in the elderly). Stronger steroid (2.5% Dermovate) can be used in the short term.
– Squamous hyperplasia: severe pruritus. Biopsy, observe and treat with topical steroids.

◆ Other vulval problems

– Lichen planus: purple/white shiny spots
– Psoriasis (rare): use moderately potent steroids as elsewhere
– Ulcers
  – herpes
  – Crohn's disease
  – chronic oral, eye and genital ulceration = Behçet's disease
  – syphilis (chancre): painless, raised, punched-out ulcer
  – tropical diseases (rare), e.g. LGV, chancroid, granuloma inguinale
– Allergy/skin irritants: ? detergents/latex (condoms)/deodorants

Swabs, skin scrapings (?fungal) may help.

◆ Vulval carcinoma

– elderly, over 70 years
– often associated epithelial changes
– 85% are squamous
– bilateral lesions occur
– check cervix for CIN or carcinoma
– spread is lymphatic to superficial inguinal, femoral or iliac nodes

Note: Melanoma/other rare skin tumours can present on the vulva.

Staging (at surgery)

0 carcinoma-in-situ
I tumour <2 cm
II tumour >2 cm

III   any size tumour with unilateral groin nodes or spread to lower vagina/urethra/anus

IV(a) involvement of upper urethra or vagina, rectal mucosa, pelvic side wall or bilateral nodes

IV(b) distant spread including to pelvic nodes

Management/ prognosis

Treatment is surgical, aiming to remove sufficient tissue to prevent local recurrence. Involves bilateral inguinal lymphadenectomy to stage and remove nodes containing tumour.

Triple incision (vulva and both groins) is just as effective and heals better than radical en-bloc excision. Well-localised lesions <2 cm can be treated by wide local excision with unilateral node dissection. Local recurrence is uncommon after radical vulvectomy (7%) with proper wide local excision.

5-year survival with negative nodes is 90% for all stages. With positive nodes it falls to 55%. Depth of invasion is indicative of node involvement: <1 mm, nodes rarely involved; 1–3 mm, groin nodes positive in 8%.

Chemotherapy (5-fluorouracil) is good for women where complete surgical resection is not an option.

◆ Vaginal discharge

Vaginal secretions during the reproductive years are normally acidic and protective. Oestrogens increase the glycogen content of vaginal squames and the commensal lactobacilli metabolise the glycogen to acid. This protective acidity is less before puberty and after the menopause, and decreased by the use of broad-spectrum antibiotics, vaginal douches or excessive cervical discharge.

Vaginal discharge is a common complaint. Over 80% of cases are physiological or due to candidiasis or trichomoniasis.

Clinically there are three situations:
1. Physiological.
2. Specific infection (trichomoniasis, candidiasis, gonorrhoea, gardnerella).
3. Mucopurulent or blood-stained.

The diagnosis is usually obvious from the history:
– colour, smell, itchiness, soreness
– sudden (infection), any urine infection?
– symptoms in the partner – ? contraception
– pill, antibiotics, steroids (candida)
– douches, pessaries, condoms (sensitivity)
– recent delivery or abortion

Increased physiological discharge (leucorrhoea) causes no odour or itch, though it may stain slightly. Unlike other causes, it contains no pus cells. It can increase due to:
– vaginal transudate (sexual excitement)
– cervical erosion (pill, pregnancy)
– ovulatory cascade of cervical mucus
– tail of IUD

If there is pus or blood, consider:
- vaginitis (atrophic, foreign body, tampon or ring pessary)
  salpingitis
- endometritis (i.e. puerperal sepsis)
- carcinoma or polyp

Management
1. Examine the abdomen for tenderness/fever (salpingitis).
2. Note any vulvitis. Pass a speculum, inspect the cervix and take a smear. Check for foreign body (e.g. retained tampon). If gonorrhoea is suspected, take swabs from urethra and cervix into Stuart's medium. Otherwise take an ordinary HVS. Take specific chlamydial swabs – endocervix, urethra and rectum. If result positive, trace contacts.
3. Perform a bimanual examination.
4. Chronic cervicitis can be treated by cryocautery, covered with antibiotic prophylaxis. Any persistent unexplained discharge is an indication for hysteroscopy and curettage.
5. In a postmenopausal woman, a bloodstained discharge is an indication for hysteroscopy and endometrial sampling/curettage to exclude endometrial carcinoma – even if there is atrophic vaginitis as a more obvious cause.
6. In a child, the combination of an under-oestrogenised vagina and poor hygiene may cause a bacterial infection. History or examination, if possible, may suggest a foreign body and EUA (using a nasal speculum or a hysteroscope passed through the opening in the hymen) may be needed to remove it.
7. Frequently no cause is found but the patient continues to complain of symptoms. Explanation about physiological discharge and avoidance of 'blind' use of antibiotics or antifungals is advised.
8. Aci-Jel pessaries may be helpful in the short term by altering vaginal pH and restoring normal flora.
9. Topical products with povidone-iodine (Betadine) are effective against candida, trichomonas, and mixed anaerobic infections: pessaries, gel or douches are available.

◆ Candidiasis (thrush)

Candida albicans is a gut commensal and should not be present in the vagina. *Predisposing factors* to vaginal candidiasis are:
    the pill
- pregnancy
- broad-spectrum antibiotics
- steroids and immunosuppression
- diabetes

The *clinical features* are itching, soreness, dyspareunia, redness and a thick white discharge with white curds (acidic). On VE grey/white patches may be seen on erythematous areas. The infection can be symptomless, especially in men. Other vaginal infection is almost invariably present and should be treated.

Treatment
- *Topical imidazole derivatives*: as cream or pessaries in 3–14 day courses. Relapse is often associated with not completing the full

course. 1-day pessary treatments are effective with good compliance (Canestan combi = clotrimazole 500 mg pessary + 2% cream, Gyno-Pevaryl 1 = econazole nitrate 150 mg, clotrimazole 500 mg pessary, Gyno-Daktarin 1 = miconazole nitrate 1.2 g)
- *Nystatin*: pessaries are effective but need a 14-day course, and preparation stains underwear
- *Oral triazole antifungals*: fluconazole (Diflucan 1) 150 mg single-dose capsule; or itraconazole (Sporanox), 1-day treatment of 400 mg b.d.

Many of these treatments are available to patients over the counter.

Antifungal cream with steroid (e.g. Canestan-HC = 1% clotrimazole + 1% hydrocortisone) is useful if there is much associated vulval inflammation. Other remedies include topical live yoghurt, homeopathy, general measures, e.g. cotton underwear, avoiding bath foams and sprays.

Topical (but not oral) therapy is safe in pregnancy.

Management of recurrent thrush
- exclude diabetes
- treat the partner (the balanitis can be symptomless)
- prophylaxis if antibiotics are prescribed with the pill
- regular prophylaxis (e.g. pessaries mid-cycle)
- systemic therapy in systemic candidiasis, or immunocompromised or HIV patients. **Note**: not recommended in pregnancy or with liver disease. There is a 1 in 10 000 chance of fatal drug-induced hepatitis, especially with ketoconazole (Nizoral).

◆ Trichomoniasis

Trichomoniasis vaginalis is a flagellate protozoan that is acquired sexually. It can cause a profuse frothy green discharge, pruritus, soreness, dyspareunia (sometimes dysuria) and intense inflammation. However, like thrush, it can be completely symptomless. The urinary tract is usually colonised as well. It can be *diagnosed* by:
- swab and culture
- cervical smear (the protozoa are also stained)
- microscopy of a drop of discharge in saline (the organisms resemble the leucocytes but are motile)

Treatment is with metronidazole (Flagyl) 400 mg b.d. for 7 days or a single dose of 2 g orally. The partner must be treated simultaneously. Alcohol must be avoided during treatment (headache, flushing, vomiting, hypotension).

◆ Gardnerella and bacterial vaginosis

(Previously called *Haemophilus vaginalis*.)
- fishy odour
- alkaline pH
- frequent carriage and asymptomatic
- associated with preterm labour

Treatment – 2% clindamycin cream (Dalacin), 5 g via applicator for 3–7 nights. Vaginal cream is safe in pregnancy. (**Note**: *systemic* clindamycin has serious side-effects, including colitis, especially in older women or after surgery.)
– metronidazole, oral or vaginal gel (Flagyl). *Not in pregnancy*
– Sultrin cream (= sulfathiazole + sulfacetamide + sulphabenzamide cream), often used following cervical cautery or surgery but *not safe in pregnancy*

Other organisms (Bacteroides, Ureaplasma, mixed anaerobes) respond to the same measures.

◆ Benign cervical conditions

1. The squamo-columnar (S–C) junction can become everted due to differential growth stimulated by oestrogens (puberty, pregnancy and the pill). The columnar epithelium becomes visible, causing the common 'erosion' (the true name is *ectropion*). 50% of women on the pill have ectropion, but treatment by cryocautery is only necessary if it is causing a symptomatic discharge, and this is often only temporarily effective.
2. The exposed columnar epithelium undergoes metaplasia to squamous epithelium and the S–C junction moves back into the canal. *Nabothian cysts*, which resemble tiny sebaceous cysts, can occur where this squamous metaplasia has blocked underlying mucosal crypts.
3. Nabothian cysts can become secondarily infected with mixed organisms, leading to *chronic cervicitis* with discharge, dyspareunia and sometimes pain. Antibiotics are usually ineffective and, providing smears are normal, treatment is by outpatient cryocautery, which takes about 10 minutes and does not require anaesthesia. It will cause a watery discharge for 2–3 weeks.
4. A *cervical polyp* can cause non-menstrual bleeding, but is often an incidental finding at smear test. If the pedicle is visible it can be twisted off, but should be sent for histology. Recurrence is less common if removed with cautery to the base, e.g. in hysteroscopy clinic setting.

◆ Cervical smears

The effectiveness of the cervical screening programme depends on the identification and treatment of CIN III (based on the assumption that carcinoma-in-situ progresses eventually to invasive carcinoma of the cervix). There are many recorded cases of this happening and pre-malignant changes are usually seen surrounding an invasive carcinoma. There is no doubt, however, that not *all* lesions progress. Factors which might indicate a greater chance of progression include heavy smoking and HPV infection.

Screening is monitored by the National Health Service Cervical Screening Programme. Standards for colposcopy clinics have also been published by this group. Among screened women, the treatment of preinvasive changes has undoubtedly reduced the incidence of invasive carcinoma. **Note**: Women at highest risk tend to be the least likely to come forward for screening.

Routine smears should be done every 3 years in all sexually active women (most programmes advocate all women between 20 and 65 years). Over 65 do a smear if they have never had one. Smear high-risk groups (STD, recurrent TOP, HPV cases) more frequently. Always inspect the cervix, because a necrotic tumour can give a negative result. About 1 in 10 cases of carcinoma-in-situ are missed (false negatives) but by repeating the first smear at 1 year this is reduced to 1 in 100.

Taking a smear
- expose the whole cervix
- sample through 360° using a wooden or plastic spatula at the squamo-columnar junction
- spread the smear immediately onto a clean, labelled glass slide
- fix immediately (do not allow to air-dry)
- complete details on request form, noting O/C, HRT, LMP

Note: The smear may be unsatisfactory if blood/polymorphs are present.

Smear results
The cytologist examines the size of the nuclei and the nuclear/cytoplasmic ratio after staining. Normal cells develop a smaller nucleus as they migrate up from the basal layer. Abnormal cells have a larger nucleus, irregular shape and may show mitoses (epithelial turnover increases and causes immature cells with larger nuclei or frank malignancy to reach the surface).

Results are expressed as *Codes*. Suggested action:
1. *Unsatisfactory* – repeat.
2. *Negative* – recall at 3-year intervals.
   There may be *Actinomyces, Trichomonas*, bacteria or *Candida* present – the report will still be 'negative'. Treat any genuine infection.
3. *Mild dyskaryosis* – repeat at 3–6 months.
   Some labs recommend colposcopy if 2nd smear is Code 3; others advise repeat at 1 year, only refering if still Code 3 then.
4. *Severe dyskaryosis* – refer for colposcopy.
5. *Severe dyskaryosis? invasive* – urgent colposcopy.
6. *? Glandular neoplasia (severe dyskaryosis with features suggesting adenocarcinoma; endocervical, endometrial or elsewhere)* – urgent referral.
7. *Moderate dyskaryosis* – refer for colposcopy.
8. *Borderline nuclear changes* – repeat at 6 months.

Borderline smears should be referred if persistent.

Severity of dyskaryosis reflects the degree of the CIN, but the match is not exact – CIN III can be found when the smear is only Code 3. Moderate dyskaryosis (Code 4) or worse usually indicates at least CIN II.

HPV infection may cause borderline nuclear changes and is often seen with mild or moderate dyskaryosis. HPV is known to be a factor in the pathogenesis of cervical cancer, but the mechanism is unknown.

Smoking and HIV infection hamper the ability of the body's natural defences to eradicate the HPV infection. Carriage rates in 20–30-year-olds are as high as 20% in studies. HPV detection on smears has been suggested as a new form of screening in the future but its role has not yet been established.

The cervical screening programme has resulted in significant falls in the death rate from cancer of the cervix. Many women over 35 (known to be the group at most risk of progression to invasive disease) are still being missed, however.

Note: A systematic computerised recall system and age/sex register is fundamental to a successful screening programme.

◆ Colposcopy and CIN

Until the mid-1970s the standard treatment for cervical intraepithelial neoplasia (CIN) was cone biopsy. The colposcope was pioneered by Stafl in the United States. In 1982 the RCOG concluded that 'ideally no patient with a CIN should be treated unless there has been prior colposcopic assessment'. In conjunction with ablative methods of treatment, the colposcope allows patients to be diagnosed and treated as outpatients with few complications.

Colposcopy:
- determines the site of lesion, particularly its upper extent
- determines whether the lesion extends to the vagina
- permits directed biopsies to be taken (some appearances are characteristic but histology is always performed)
- is fundamental to all the local destructive techniques

Since CIN does not show 'skip' lesions, the whole area can be assessed (unlike VIN).

The colposcope is a microscope with a powerful light source mounted on a stand. The cervix is exposed with a bivalve speculum with the patient in lithotomy position. The cervix is wiped with normal saline. Abnormal epithelium may appear a deeper pink than the normal pale pink squamous epithelium. Next the cervix is painted with 5% acetic acid which is a protein coagulant that stains abnormal immature epithelium white (because immature cells have less glycogen and more cytoplasmic protein). The degree of whiteness of the demarcated area and the coarseness of the vascular pattern visible in the underlying strata, either as dots (punctate) or as a network (mosaic) allows an estimate of the degree of CIN present. A directed biopsy is taken and local destruction therapy applied then or later after histology results are known.

The presence of large atypical vessels (corkscrew or right-angled bifurcations) is associated with invasive foci and indicates the need for a deeper biopsy. In cases where the lesion extends out of sight into the endocervical canal or where the whole S–C junction is not visible, its full extent cannot be assessed and loop excision for histological assessment is recommended. True surgical cone biopsy is rarely indicated since wide loop excision is often enough to assess depth of invasion to plan surgery.

The *histology* of the biopsy is reported as:
- CIN I
- CIN II
- CIN III
- Micro-invasion
- Frank invasion

◆ Ablative methods of treatment for CIN

All methods aim for effective destruction of abnormal areas with minimal risk to fertility. They include:
- diathermy (loop excision or deep needle)
- cold coagulation
- laser
- cryocautery (for mildest lesions only)

There has recently been a report of suspected cell survival after cryocautery. The area treated by laser or diathermy loop excision heals completely after 1 month and there is appreciably less discomfort and vaginal discharge. One advantage of the colposcope is that if the transformation zone extends out onto the vaginal wall (about 4% of women) it can be identified and destroyed.

Complications of cervical treatments:
- infection and haemorrhage
- cervical incompetence (especially cone biopsy, up to 25%)
- cervical stenosis (rare)
- infertility (loss of cervical mucus, sequel to infection)

Follow-up smears are essential and if they become abnormal further biopsy is indicated. Suspicious areas can be followed up by repeat colposcopy.

◆ Carcinoma of the cervix

On average, a GP will see carcinoma of the cervix about once every 5 years. Most women are over 40 but the incidence in younger women is rising. The cause seems to be related to coitus and to early age of first coitus. Other associations are probably secondary to this. It is extremely rare in virgins and is associated with:
- early sex
- smoking
- HPV infection
- high parity
- low socioeconomic group
- multiple partners
- other STD

The carcinogenic agent was originally thought to be Herpes virus type 2 or sperm DNA but in 1976 an association was noted with wart virus infection. Human papillomavirus DNA has been identified in cervical cancer tissue and particular types are firmly associated with the cancer.

Micro-invasive carcinoma causes no signs or symptoms. Once invasive, *the classical symptom is non-menstrual bleeding*, which may be:
– postcoital (ALWAYS SUSPECT THE CERVIX)
– intermenstrual
– postmenopausal

Pain, discharge, fistulae and uraemia are all late features.

Staging and treatment

The tumour is staged clinically (Table 1). This involves:
– EUA and biopsy
– rectal examination (?parametrial involvement)
– cystoscopy (?bladder involvement)
   (CT scan of the pelvis and the subsequent surgery do not form part of the staging.)

95% of cervical cancer is squamous carcinoma. *Lymph node involvement depends on the depth of invasion.*
– invasion < 1 mm: the chance of positive nodes is negligible
– 1–3 mm invasion: risk is 1%. For lesions <3 mm depth and <7 mm across (stage 1a^1) cone biopsy may be adequate and hysterectomy may be avoided (retains fertility)
– 3–5 mm invasion: risk is 4% – advise hysterectomy with lymphadenectomy

For stage 1b, survival depends on the *type* of surgery offered – it is greater when more radical surgery is done and when nodes are taken.

For stages 1b, 2a and 2b, the survival is the same after primary surgical or primary radiotherapy management, but the *complications* are different. Choose the method of treatment depending the patient's circumstances. Primary surgery provides histological information on node status. Radiotherapy can be intra-cavity (caesium) or external.

For advanced disease (stage 3 or 4), treat with radiotherapy $\pm$ chemotherapy.

Radiotherapy complications include:
– vaginal stenosis (preventable by regular intercourse)
– haematuria (bladder telangiectasia)
– cystitis
– vesico-vaginal fistula (6 months later)
– ureteric fibrosis and obstruction
– adhesions

Pelvic exenteration is used for *recurrent disease*. 5-year survival can be 50% and the surgical morbidity is surprisingly low (< 5%).

Surgery is the treatment of choice for *adenocarcinoma*.

Advanced disease

Terminal problems associated with advanced disease include:
– pain
– bleeding
– infection (vaginal erosion)
– fistulae
– gut obstruction
– ureteric obstruction

Death is due to renal failure (50%), anaemia, infection or cachexia.

Table 1 Clinical staging of carcinoma cervix

Stage	Spread	Primary treatment	Approx. 5-yr survival (%)
0	Carcinoma in situ (CIN III)		
1	Confined to the uterus		70–90 (more for 1a^1)
1a	Invasive cancer only identifiable microscopically 1a^1: invasion ⩽ 3 mm depth and lesion ⩽ 7 mm width 1a^2: invasion ⩾ 3 mm but ⩽ 5 mm, and ⩽ 7 mm width	Cone excision or hysterectomy Wider excision hysterectomy (remove also medial 1/2 cardinal and uterosacral ligaments) + lymphadenectomy	Surgery*
1b	Larger than 1a 1b^1: tumour < 4 cm 1b^2: tumour ⩾ 4 cm		
2	Invading beyond the uterus but not to pelvic side wall or lower 1/3 vagina	Wertheim's hysterectomy + lymphadenectomy ± removal of suspicious para-aortic nodes	70
2a	Upper 2/3 vagina, no parametrial invasion		
2b	With parametrial invasion but not out to pelvic side wall		
3	Extending to side wall and/or lower 1/3 vagina and/or hydronephrosis or non-functioning kidney	Radiotherapy	40
3a	To lower 1/3 vagina		
3b	To side wall or hydronephrosis or non-functioning kidney		
4	Invades mucosa of bladder or rectum and/or extends beyond true pelvis		15 (less for 4b)
4a	Invading bladder or rectum		
4b	Distant spread	Palliative care	

Note: Tumours > 4 cm are difficult to excise with clear margins and have high incidence of regional node metastasis so primary surgery is less favoured.

◆ Pelvic inflammatory disease

Pelvic sepsis may be acute or chronic, is debilitating and adversely affects future fertility. Proper accurate diagnosis is essential – over-diagnosis is common in the GP setting and leads to multiple speculative courses of antibiotics over a prolonged period. Acute disease merits accurate diagnosis in hospital and may require i.v. antibiotics.

Acute salpingitis

The important associations are:
– puerperal or post-abortal ($\pm$ anaerobes)
– IUD in situ
– gonococcal
– chlamydial
– iatrogenic (failure of prophylaxis for pelvic procedures or investigations)

Sepsis arises due to ascending infection and therefore is not seen in pregnancy after 12 weeks when the decidual membranes seal off the tubes. It is always bilateral although symptoms may appear unilateral.

The patient is acutely unwell with:
– bilateral pain and tenderness, sometimes with upper quadrant pain due to perihepatic involvement (esp. chlamydia)
– dyspareunia
– fever
– vomiting
– vaginal discharge
– marked pelvic tenderness (on moving the cervix and in the fornices)
– urinary symptoms

Urethral and cervical swabs should always be taken to exclude gonorrhoea. HVS is often negative however, and peritoneal swabs taken at laparoscopy (for both aerobic and anaerobic culture) are needed. *Diagnostic laparoscopy* is necessary to confirm the situation (clinical impression is wrong in one-third of cases) especially for the first attack or to distinguish from ectopic pregnancy (urinary or serum β-HCG helpful). *Differential diagnosis* includes appendicitis, endometriosis, ectopic pregnancy, ovarian cyst accidents and corpus luteum bleeding. Laparoscopy is also indicated for any episode where the woman is acutely ill and fails to respond rapidly to broad-spectrum antibiotics (always including drugs against chlamydia). Pelvic abscess requires surgical drainage. In older women pelvic or gut malignancy and diverticular abscess must be excluded.

Note: Acute chlamydial infection can present with right upper quadrant pain due to perihepatic adhesions (Fitz-Hugh-Curtis syndrome).

Treatment

Drug treatment regimens must cover chlamydia, gonococcus and anaerobes, to reduce tubal damage and subsequent infertility. USA research trials confirm the following regimens to be of proven effectiveness:
1. *Either* cefoxitin 2 g i.v. q.d.s. in acute phase (or single dose 2 g i.m. with probenecid), *or* clindamycin 900 mg i.v. t.d.s. + gentamicin 2 mg/kg stat reducing to 1.5 mg/kg t.d.s. after 48 hrs, with doxycycline 100 mg orally b.d. for at least 14 days.

2. *For outpatients*: ofloxacin 400 mg stat, followed by 14 days oral treatment with *either* clindamycin 450 mg q.d.s. or metronidazole 500 mg b.d.

An IUD should be removed and submitted for microbiological analysis. Contact tracing and treatment is essential. Most GU clinics have good contact-tracing systems and referral is advised, especially for chlamydia and gonorrhoea. Blood tests for chlamydial antibodies are available but not much used acutely. In pregnancy, inform paediatricians if mother known to be a carrier at delivery.

Complications
- infertility: tubal damage 10–15% after one episode; 75% after three
- tubal abscess (surgical drainage required)
- subsequent ectopic pregnancy
- chronic pelvic pain

Chronic salpingitis
- recurrent acute salpingitis
- tuberculosis
- *ureaplasma/mycoplasma* particularly implicated in chronic infection

The tubes become occluded, fibrous adhesions develop and the uterus is fixed in retroversion. The *symptoms* are:
- pain (congestive dysmenorrhoea, deep dyspareunia, low abdominal and back pain)
- menorrhagia
- discharge and low-grade fever
- bilateral tender adnexal masses

There is often a history of previous attacks of salpingitis but laparoscopy may be necessary to differentiate it from endometriosis. Acute exacerbations are common and prolonged courses of rotating antibiotics are necessary. If it is causing chronic ill-health, hysterectomy and bilateral salpingectomy is the best treatment, conserving healthy ovarian tissue if possible.

Pelvic tuberculosis
Always due to haematogenous spread. Usually presents with infertility but can produce all the above symptoms and mimic chronic pelvic sepsis. It is suspected if there is a history of contact/travel, if the patient is a virgin or if there is no response to antibiotics. CXR, ESR and lymphocyte counts would be indicated but the definitive diagnosis is on histology of curettings. *Treatment* is in two stages, best supervised in a hospital setting.
- Initial phase: minimum 2 months combined therapy with 3–4 drugs (rifampicin + pyrazinamide + isoniazid + ethambutol if resistance likely)
- Continuation phase: further 4 months using rifampicin + isoniazid

Anti-infective agents in acute pelvic inflammatory disease

For chlamydia:
Tetracyclines are effective but unsuitable in pregnancy or while breastfeeding.
- *doxycycline*: oral, 100 mg b.d. for 7–21 days (give for 21 days in pelvic inflammatory disease)

Macrolides
- *erythromycin:* 50 mg/kg/day by i.v. infusion

- *azithromycin*: oral, 1 g as single dose or 500 mg daily for 3 days (Zithromax)

Quinolones
- *ciprofloxacin*: oral, 250–500 mg as single dose; i.v. 100 mg single dose (Ciproxin)
- *ofloxacin:* oral 400 mg single dose (Tarivid)

For N. gonorrhoeae:
Although often effective, in many areas *N. gonorrhoeae* is no longer reliably sensitive to penicillins such as co-amoxiclav (Augmentin), and this is no longer the drug of choice.

Second and third generation cephalosporins are highly effective: many can be used as a single dose, especially useful for outpatients and contacts.
- *cefuroxime*: i.v. 750 mg–1.5 g t.d.s. or q.d.s.; i.m. 1.5 g single dose (give divided between 2 sites) (Zinacef)
- *cefuroxime axetil*: oral, 1 g single dose (Zinnat)
- *cefotaxime*: i.v. 1 g single dose (Claforan)
- *ceftriaxone*: i.m. 250 mg single dose (Rocephin)

◆ Pelvic mass

Often an incidental finding at smear check or ultrasound for pregnancy. A lump in the pelvis is notoriously difficult to diagnose clinically. A malignant ovarian tumour is always a possibility. The possibilities are:
   ovarian cyst or tumour
- fibroid (especially if pedunculated)
- full bladder
   early pregnancy
- ectopic pregnancy
- endometriosis (chocolate cysts)
- hydro/pyo-salpinx
- bowel (faeces, diverticular disease, carcinoma, Crohn's)
- pelvic kidney (very rare)
- haematocolpos (pubertal girls)

Note: Ultrasound can distinguish: pregnancy, normal ovaries separate from the mass, associated fluid in the POD, liver metastases, normal kidneys, cystic *vs* solid nature of the lesion. It cannot tell you the diagnosis nor the histology. Vaginal ultrasound is especially useful, does not require a full bladder and is well tolerated by patients.

◆ Fibroids

Fibroids are benign tumours (leiomyomata) of the uterine smooth muscle and are often multiple. They may grow inwards (submucous) or outwards (subserous) and are often asymptomatic. They enlarge in pregnancy, on the pill or with HRT, due to oestrogen stimulation, and regress after the menopause. They are more common in Africans, often presenting in young women.

Signs and symptoms:
- menorrhagia
- pressure (frequency, dyspareunia)

- abdominal mass
- ? infertility (unproven)

Ultrasound confirms the diagnosis and excludes ovarian cyst.

Complications:
- hyaline degeneration (asymptomatic)
- torsion of pedunculated fibroid
- malignant change (very rare – MRI helpful)
- in pregnancy:
    - fetal malpresentation (often leads to difficult caesarean section)
    - red degeneration (pain, fever, vomiting) due to growth outstripping blood supply. Differential diagnosis: pain due to abruption. Conservative treatment

Treatment:
- often none required. Fibroids regress after the menopause (except on HRT)
- menorrhagia may need treatment: hysterectomy – TAH or laparoscopically-assisted vaginal hysterectomy
- myomectomy (risks: TAH if bleeding uncontrolled, scar rupture in pregnancy, tubal infertility due to adhesions)
- hysteroscopic resection of submucous fibroids with TCRE
- medical treatment (danazol, GnRH analogues) may cause regression and is useful for preparation before minimally-invasive surgical treatment. Can be used alone, especially close to the menopause.

◆ Hysterectomy

Most hysterectomies are performed for benign conditions. Each GP is likely to be involved with counselling at least two women per year for the operation. There is a low mortality and morbidity (prior anaemia) for the operation as most patients are fit. There is a wide geographical variation in hysterectomy rates – and operative route – depending on consultant preference, laparoscopic expertise and patient expectation. Nowadays alternative treatments for menorrhagia mean that far fewer hysterectomies are done for a 'normal' uterus. Laparoscopic surgery combined with a vaginal procedure offers a quicker postoperative recovery and small scars. The pelvis and abdomen can be thoroughly inspected. Increased expertise in more difficult vaginal hysterectomy (morcellation, piecemeal removal, vaginal oophorectomy) or pretreatment to 'shrink' fibroids has also reduced the number of traditional TAHs.

Vaginal hysterectomy has the following advantages over the abdominal approach:
- less postoperative bowel dysfunction
- shorter anaesthetic time and intubation/ventilation not essential
- regional anaesthesia possible
- no scar in rectus sheath
- can be combined with prolapse procedures, suspension and repairs

Prophylactic oophorectomy (+ subsequent HRT) is advocated to reduce the risk of subsequent ovarian cancer but if this were to be done in

500 procedures only 1–2 ovarian malignancies would be prevented. Depends on the patient's age, family history, contraindications to HRT, so counselling is essential. Formal genetic counselling can identify women at greater risk for ovarian cancer who should be offered prophylactic oophorectomy.

Some evidence suggests a risk of premature ovarian failure within 5 years of hysterectomy (TAH); others dispute this. The route chosen for surgery may influence this if ovarian blood supply is implicated in the aetiology.

◆ Endometriosis

A chronic scarring and adhesion-forming condition in which ectopic endometrium is found outside the uterus, usually on the ovaries and in the pouch of Douglas, but occasionally at distant sites. Pelvic disease may follow implantation of endometrium following retrograde menstruation. It bleeds at the time of menstruation, causing an intense fibrous reaction and dense adhesions. It can be symptomless even when extensive, but the typical clinical picture is of an infertile woman of 30–45 years with:
– dysmenorrhoea
– dyspareunia
– menorrhagia
– tender (fixed) retroverted uterus
– ovarian masses (chocolate cysts/adhesions)

Clinical diagnosis is difficult and laparoscopy is essential to distinguish endometriosis from chronic salpingitis. The tubes characteristically remain patent in endometriosis, although bound with adhesions, and infertility is probably due to tube–ovary–broad ligament adhesions and ovarian deposits preventing ovum release.

Endometriosis regresses if cyclical oestrogen changes are prevented (pregnancy, after the menopause, continuous O/C) and *medical treatment* is based on suppressing/abolishing this cycle.
– continous combined O/C
– GnRH analogues. Highly effective but menopausal side-effects severe. Not androgenic. Do not use for more than 6 months continuously due to osteoporosis risk of prolonged hypo-oestrogenic state. Hot flushes can be offset by low-dose clonidine or tibolone (Livial) or by 'adding back' a small transdermal oestrogen dose in months 3–6 of treatment
– danazol (unwelcome androgenic side-effects)

Drug therapy is usually insufficient for extensive disease/chocolate cysts and *surgical treatment* may be required:
– laparoscopic destruction of deposits by laser, diathermy, division of adhesions
– excision of chocolate cysts
– pelvic clearance including oophorectomy for severe pain ('frozen pelvis')
– hysterectomy alone may benefit adenomyosis (endometriosis buried within the myometrium)

◆ Ovarian cysts

May be benign or malignant, cystic or solid, unilateral or bilateral. Commonest are benign: often functional (usually small, unilocular), can be multiple. Small cystic areas up to 2.5–3 cm across are commonly seen on ultrasound scans (may be the normal cyclical workings of the ovary).

Combined oral contraceptive protects against benign cysts.

Progesterone-only pill and clomiphene – slightly increased risk.

Histology:
- follicular
- serous
- mucinous
- corpus luteum cysts
- cystic teratoma (dermoid) 20% bilateral
- theca-lutein cysts (hyperstimulation in infertility treatments, or can be multiple with hydatidiform mole)
- endometriosis (chocolate cysts)

Complications:
- torsion
- haemorrhage into the cyst
- rupture
- malignancy (always a risk unless histology known for certain)

Management:

Small (<3–4 cm) simple cysts can be managed expectantly: re-scan 3–4 months later, preferably at a different time in the cycle.

Laparoscopy – with simple drainage, cystectomy, or oophorectomy. Wedge biopsy of other ovary if histology in doubt.

Ovarian cysts in pregnancy

Can present as 'large for dates' by upward displacement of the uterus. Usually no action required if simple and small (<6 cm). Monitor by serial scans. Corpus luteum cysts regress by the second trimester. If larger or symptomatic, remove in second trimester or shortly after delivery to prevent later complications (risk of torsion in early puerperium as uterus involutes). Rarely, large cysts can cause malpresentations and obstructed labour.

◆ Malignant ovarian disease

In the UK ovarian cancer kills over 6000 women every year. It is usually diagnosed late and results in more deaths than those from cervical and uterine cancer combined. Overall 5 year survival is <50% despite aggressive therapy.

Risk is reduced by:
- sustained use of combined O/C
- having >1 live birth
- breastfeeding
- previous hysterectomy or tubal ligation (this may be related to the associated fertility of these women)
- prophylactic oophorectomy in women >40 having a hysterectomy

Use of postmenopausal HRT for >10 years slightly *increases risk*. Risk is also increased by nulliparity and with a family history (genetic referral advised for high-risk families).

Pathogenesis is unclear: some think that it may be caused by repeated ovulation disrupting the epithelial surface of the ovary; others suggest the increased risk in infertile patients is due to high resting GnRH levels, or to drug treatments given to cause ovarian stimulation (a US study showed that the relative risk after fertility drugs may be three or more times higher than controls).

Characteristics of ovarian tumours:
- cystic or solid or mixed
- 90% epithelial in origin (derived from serosa of ovary)
- relatively common – 14 in 100 000 women in the UK
- peak incidence 60–70 years
- late presentation (70% stage III or IV already) – this gives poor prognosis overall

Symptoms:
- abdominal pain/distension/mass
- weight gain (ascites, may lead to change in clothes size)
- weight loss (cachexia)
- pain is rare
- urinary obstruction
- symptoms of secondary deposits

Screening for ovarian cancer

Screening can detect ovarian cancer in asymptomatic women, leading to treatment at an earlier stage. However, there is no evidence yet that this reduces deaths. Main methods tried have been ultrasound, clinical examination and the cancer antigen 125 test (CA125).
- clinical examination: unreliable
- ultrasound: sensitivity almost 100%, but lacks specificity (false positive rate 2.5%)
- CA125: sensitivity less (80%), but more specific (false positives <1%)

Trials of screening currently underway in UK and USA. At present there is no good evidence for screening low-risk women.

High-risk women – family history, genetic (BRCA1 and 2 mutations).
- 1 affected first-degree relative: 2–3 × increased risk
- >1 affected first-degree relative: 10 × increased risk (for woman age 45 has a 10–15% chance of contracting the disease by age 75)

BRCA1 mutation occurs in 5% of women who develop ovarian cancer under age 70. It also occurs in breast cancer families. Refer to geneticist if family history suggestive.

Preoperative assessment

Note: It is important to assess *preoperatively* whether an ovarian mass is likely to be malignant – if so, surgery by gynae/oncologist gives better results than by generalist: transfer to cancer centre.

Clinical examination cannot distinguish reliably between benign and malignant masses except in advanced disease.

Malignancy is more likely if:
- age > 60 yrs
- CA125 > 35 u/ml (**Note**: CA125 also rises with active PID and endometriosis)
- ultrasound shows large mass, solid or mixed echoes, ascites

CT scan is very helpful – ascites, liver metastases, bowel involvement, bilateral tumours, renal obstruction.

Also check CXR, LFTs, U&Es and other tumour markers (HCG, LDH, AFP).

Management

Surgery always useful except in terminal cases:
- stage the tumour
- reduce tumour mass to increase the success of adjuvant therapies
- option of diversion procedure (bowel/urinary)
- reduce ascites formation by omentectomy

In young women, unilateral oophorectomy for borderline and very early invasive disease is a possible option, which has 5–10% recurrence rate. Remove remaining ovary after family complete.

Chemotherapy:
No benefit in stage I disease.

Combination regimens with platinum are best. Best triple regimens include cyclophosphamide, doxorubicin and cisplatin (CAP). Regimens with carboplatin are less toxic than cisplatin.

In advanced disease, regimens using paclitaxel (Taxol) in combination with cisplatin give, on average, an extra year's survival.

Patients who do not respond to platinum regimens may benefit from paclitaxel alone.

Radiotherapy:
No benefit over surgery in early disease.

May be of benefit as palliative treatment of advanced disease (e.g. for dyspnoea with lung metastases, vaginal and rectal bleeding, pain relief) but overall survival not improved.

Staging of ovarian cancer

Staging is done at surgery:

I – confined to ovaries
   a) one
   b) both
   c) one or both, with ascites/positive peritoneal washings

II – extension within pelvis
   a) to uterus/tubes
   b) to other pelvic organs
   c) = a) or b), with ascites or positive cytology on washing

III – extension outside the pelvis within the peritoneal cavity (including bowel or omentum)
   a) microscopic peritoneal spread (biopsies)
   b) peritoneal deposits < 2 cm
   c) deposits > 2 cm ± nodes involved

IV – distant spread, usually liver or malignant pleural effusion

Other ovarian tumours
(rare)
- germ cell tumours: benign or malignant teratomas (dermoid cysts)
- sex cord tumours: granulosa or theca cell, secrete oestrogens
- secondary tumours from other organs, particularly bowel 'Krukenberg' tumours, usually secondaries from stomach)
- endometrioid carcinoma, ?primary ovarian, ?endometrial origin
- fibromas

◆ The menopause

Defined strictly as the last occurrence of a true menstrual period. The term 'climacteric' encompasses the various changes occurring at this time. Problems are often compounded by other events going on at this stage in a woman's life (work, family, domestic changes). The average age for cessation of periods in the UK is 51 with a wide range between 40 and 57 years.

The *main immediate problems* are:
- irregular cycles with variable loss, often heavy
- hot flushes, night sweats (leading to insomnia and chronic tiredness)
- genital atrophy (dyspareunia), loss of libido
- mood changes
- deciding when to discontinue contraception

Longer-term sequelae are of concern for the individual and also from a public health/NHS resource standpoint:
- osteoporosis
- arterial disease (coronary and cerebral)
- hormone replacement therapy (HRT) – prophylaxis or therapy?

Irregular cycles:
Common as the menopause approaches because falling oestrogen levels (follicular failure) no longer stimulate an LH surge and cycles become anovulatory.

Postmenopausal bleeding:
Defined as vaginal bleeding more than 6 months after the last period, and *always warrants investigation* to exclude endometrial carcinoma. Check general health, hormone or other treatment, heaviness and pattern of bleeding, pelvic examination, smear result. (This is a good opportunity to examine the breasts also and discuss NHS programme of mammography screening.)
　　Endometrial sampling by outpatient curettage (Pipelle aspiration) and transvaginal pelvic ultrasound to assess endometrial thickness are required. If no endometrial sample is obtained and atrophic endometrium is seen on scan, reassure and stress the importance of reporting further episodes. Hysteroscopy (as an outpatient under LA, or in theatre under GA) and biopsy are essential if bleeding is recurrent or the bleeding pattern is suggestive of carcinoma (continuous blood-stained loss). A significant proportion – up to 25% – of recurrent PMB patients do have endometrial carcinoma or atypical hyperplasia, and proceeding to hysterectomy with BSO is justified even if repeat investigations fail to make the diagnosis.

Simple endometrial hyperplasia without atypia responds to high-dose oral progestogens – repeat histology after 3 months of treatment is essential; if atypia persists (rare), hysterectomy is advised.

Contraception:
Barrier methods, the POP or the IUD can be stopped 12 months after the last period. If there is amenorrhoea and hot flushes, it can be assumed that fertility has ceased.

The POP is very effective at this stage of relatively low fertility (failure rate about 0.5%) and it often helps hot flushes. However, if breakthrough bleeding occurs, curettage is necessary.

In the absence of smoking, obesity or hypertension, it may be more acceptable to continue the combined pill (no more than 35 µg oestrogen) up to the menopause. HRT is *not* contraceptive.

Vasomotor instability:
Causes hot flushes with sweating and palpitations. They occur in 75% but only about 15% request treatment. Attacks last a few minutes and can occur up to several times an hour. They may continue for a few months or for 5 years or more but eventually cease even without treatment. They are probably due to high FSH levels and respond within days to oestrogen given as HRT. If oestrogens are contraindicated low-dose clonidine or tibolone is useful. Progesterone treatment may help but the mechanism is unclear.

Genital tract atrophy:
Predisposes to:
– atrophic vaginitis
– prolapse
– stress incontinence and urgency

Atrophic vaginitis is common, causing soreness, dysuria, dyspareunia and eventually shrinkage of the introitus. There may be bloodstained discharge (often sterile but as there is a tendency to bacterial infection because of loss of protective acidity, therefore take swabs).

Atrophy is treated with topical oestrogens (e.g. cream, pessaries or Estring), or with oral or transdermal preparations. Unopposed oestrogens (by any route) should *never* be used in women with a uterus. If oestrogens are contraindicated, non-hormonal preparations such as vaginal lubricants or hygroscopic preparations may help with dyspareunia and dryness.

Mood changes:
Headaches, insomnia (often due to sweats and flushes), irritability and depression are common around the menopause. Often they are due to simultaneous stresses associated with family and job, together with feelings of loss of attractiveness and low self-esteem. Oestrogen deficiency does cause mood changes, however, and these respond dramatically to HRT. Clinical depression is better treated with a tricyclic antidepressant which also helps the patient to sleep or one of the SSRI preparations, although these lack the sedative effect and can exacerbate insomnia.

Osteoporosis/fractures:
The incidence of these conditions increases dramatically in women not taking oestrogens, especially fractured neck of femur or wrist and crush fractures of the vertebrae. Morbidity and mortality are significant. The cost to the NHS of treating such fractures easily outweighs the cost of universal HRT. This can be used as an argument for prolonged HRT, a topic with major financial implications and epidemiological significance.

Hip fractures:
- lifetime risk is 15% for a 50-year-old Caucasian female (>30% for vertebral fracture)
- 25% die within 12 months of the fracture
- at least 50% lose mobility and cannot return to previous activities

By age 75, 50% of all women will have had hip, wrist or spinal fractures.

Myocardial infarction, cardiovascular and lipid changes:
Plasma cholesterol, triglycerides and VLDL rise and HDL falls, increasing risk for ischaemic heart disease. Epidemiology confirms rises in IHD in postmenopausal women and in early menopause or oophorectomy patients. At 50 years, women have a low risk of IHD, but, by age 80, the risk is the same for men and women.

Hormone replacement therapy (HRT)

Indications:
- symptomatic relief
- prophylaxis (against osteoporosis/IHD (?, trials ongoing)/and Alzheimer's disease)

Check there are no *contraindications:*
- breast cancer
- thromboembolic disorders
- oestrogen-dependent tumours
- liver disease
- combination of several milder factors (e.g. obesity, smoking, hypertension)

If there is no uterus, continuous unopposed oestrogens are safe. If the uterus is intact, this would cause endometrial hyperplasia and malignancy, so oppose with at least 12 days progestogen each month. *Combined formulations* avoid the patient deliberately omitting the additional progestogens. Transdermal oestrogens are the most physiological route, permitting very low dosage as there is no initial metabolism in the liver. Change twice weekly. Use the lowest effective dose. Combination patches are now available.

Long-term cyclical HRT is less popular now: women on these preparations will continue to have bleeds and find less relief from flushes etc. when the progestogen component is added.

Continuous combined forms of HRT avoid the withdrawal bleeding that many older women find unacceptable (especially if they also have atrophic vaginitis). It should not usually be started until after menopause has been confirmed (by FSH). For premenopausal symptom relief, start with opposed regimens.

In the USA many women continue to receive unopposed oestrogens but undergo annual curettage to check histology. Prolonged unopposed oestrogens, even transdermally, are unwise, however, as endometrial stimulation occurs due to good systemic absorption, especially through atrophic skin.

Progestogen compliance is difficult with *oestrogen implants*, requiring tablet opposition by progestogens on a regular cyclical basis, and implants are best reserved for hysterectomised women for this reason. Tachyphylaxis is said not to be a problem if 50 mg (not 100 mg) implants are used. There is no value in measuring serum oestrogen levels in terms of assessing the frequency of replacement implants, although some specialists refuse repeat implants if levels are persistently high.

Note: Combination HRT entails two prescription charges for the patient!

Erratic bleeding on HRT requires investigation. HRT is *not* a contraceptive (the dose of oestrogen is only equivalent to about 10 μg of the synthetic oestrogen used in the combined pill).

Most patients continue treatment for 2–5 years. Withdrawal bleeding is the commonest reason for stopping therapy. For bone prophylaxis, continue for 5–10 years. (Osteoclast activity is reduced, new bone is not made.) Other measures are important in reducing osteoporosis risk: stopping smoking, diet, exercise, thyroid disease. HRT need not be stopped before major elective surgery, provided perioperative thromboprophylaxis is used.

Tibolone (Livial) Has oestrogenic, progestogenic and weak androgenic activity. Do not use before the menopause. May precipitate irregular bleeding if started within 1 year of the last period. After this women usually stay without periods. Indicated for treatment of hot flushes and for prophylaxis against osteoporosis – give continuously (2.5 mg daily) without breaks. Is licensed for 'add-back' therapy to prevent vasomotor symptoms associated with GnRH analogue treatment (e.g. for endometriosis) in premenopausal women.

Selective oestrogen receptor modulators (SERMs) These will become more popular as they have beneficial oestrogen effects on bone and on coronary artery disease, without the stimulating effects on endometrium and breast. (Earlier examples with different effects and uses from oestrogens were clomiphene and tamoxifen.) The first second-generation SERM available on prescription is raloxifene, currently licensed for the prevention of vertebral fractures in postmenopausal women at *high* risk of osteoporosis. It does not seem to cause endometrial pathology and reduces LDL-cholesterol. It should not be used to control hot flushes (convential HRT is advised). The risk of DVT on treatment is increased – until RCT data are available, stop raloxifene before elective surgery.

Expect this treatment to be licensed soon for prevention and treatment of osteoporosis in low-risk women too. May also reduce breast cancer risk, especially the third-generation SERMs now under development.

Disodium etidronate (Didronel PMO)

90-day cycles of treatment with disodium etidronate (a bisphosphonate) for 14 days, then calcium carbonate for 76 days. Licensed for prevention and treatment of osteoporosis, particularly useful if oestrogens cannot be given.

◆ Endometrial carcinoma

On average a GP will see one new case every 7 years. Eight out of ten cases occur postmenopausally: the peak age is 60 years; it is rare below 35 years. The usual presenting symptom is postmenopausal bleeding (PMB). 50% of pyometra cases have underlying endometrial malignancy.

Risk factors include nulliparity, obesity, diabetes and prolonged use of unopposed oestrogens. It is also more common in women with high resting-oestrogen levels, as in some PCO patients.

Histology: is usually *adenocarcinoma* (can be endometrioid). Adenosquamous, clear cell or papillary serous tumours have worse prognosis. Adenoacanthoma (adenocarcinoma with squamous metaplasia) has a slightly better prognosis. *Sarcomas* are rare: grade (low or high) determines prognosis. *Mixed Müllerian tumours* have epithelial and stromal elements and are rare.

Investigation of PMB

Endometrial cancer presents early with bleeding — *always* investigate (do not dismiss as atrophic change):
- smear
- endometrial histology: outpatient Pipelle biopsy is as accurate as D&C in looking for malignancy
- ultrasound (transvaginal) for endometrial thickness
- hysteroscopy

A normal ultrasound can reliably exclude endometrial cancer: the specificity depends on the cut-off used (e.g. 4 or 6 mm) when measuring endometrial thickness. Outpatient hysteroscopy is safe, reduces the number of admissions and general anaesthetics and is acceptable to most women.

Note: Repeated PMB is suspicious of malignancy even if biopsies have failed to diagnose it.

Staging and prognosis

Staging of endometrial cancer is surgical:

Ia – limited to endometrium
Ib – invasion of < 1/2 depth of myometrium
Ic – invasion of > 1/2 depth of myometrium

IIa – to endocervical glands
IIb – to cervical stroma

IIIa – to adnexae or to serosal surface of uterus (± positive peritoneal washings)

IIIb – pelvic or para-aortic nodes

IVa – invasion of bowel or bladder
IVb – distant spread $\pm$ inguinal or intra-abdominal nodes

The 'curable' nature of early endometrial cancer has been questioned – a significant number of stage I cases (10–20%) will have node involvement. Overall 5 year survival of stage I disease is 70%; for stage II it is less than 60%.

MRI scan preoperatively can help to assess nodes and the extent of myometrial invasion or cervical involvement.

Treatment Treatment of early disease is *surgical*, although radiotherapy is as effective (but has more side-effects). Lymphadenectomy or node sampling improves prognosis, probably because the stage is not then underestimated.

Chemotherapy: high dose progestogens have no benefit in primary disease. Progestogens, tamoxifen and platinum/paclitaxel regimens have been tried in recurrent disease but there is no proven survival benefit.

Radiotherapy: as adjunctive therapy after surgery (vault or external pelvic) irradiation reduces pelvic recurrence. No proven effect on survival.

Most vault recurrence occurs in the first year but lifelong follow-up is required as metastatic relapse may be late, to lung, bone, vagina or inguinal nodes.

◆ Genital tract prolapse

The main associations are pregnancy and vaginal delivery, menopausal atrophy and raised intra-abdominal pressure (e.g. obesity, smoker's cough or rarely ascites or a large ovarian cyst). It is sometimes seen in the nulliparous, however, presumably due to a congenital weakness of the main uterine supports (transverse cervical and uterosacral ligaments) that normally anchor the cervix in the middle of the pelvis.

The diagnostic pointer in the history is that all the *symptoms* are worse on standing and relieved by lying down:
– 'something coming down'
– backache
– stress incontinence

The patient may also complain of difficulty in voiding urine or defaecating, which they relieve by digital pressure on either the anterior or posterior vaginal wall.

Assessment: The diagnosis is confirmed by examination (standing, ideally!). Prolapsed vaginal wall (cystocele, rectocele) can occur without uterine descent but prolapse of the uterus (descent of the cervix below the level of the ischial spines) rarely occurs alone.

The left lateral position, using a Sims speculum to retract the perineum, is the best position to demonstrate a prolapse. Uterine descent is best assessed by bimanual examination or by using a tenaculum on the cervix to draw the uterus gently downwards.

Grade I   – uterine descent into vagina
Grade II   – descent to the introitus
Grade III – cervix protrudes beyond introitus
Grade IV – uterus completely outside the vagina (procidentia). Ureters may become obstructed and are a hazard at surgery due to their lower position.

Distinguish also between urethrocele, cystocele, enterocele and rectocele. A PR is helpful.

Treatment

1. A polyethylene *ring pessary* (rubber ones can cause vaginitis): this is inserted like a diaphragm and should be changed every 4 months. There is often an element of atrophy, when oestrogens are helpful. The woman should be encouraged to lose weight and stop smoking.

   A pessary can be used if the woman is unfit for surgery or is awaiting surgery. A pessary can also be used in early pregnancy if there is any prolapse and removed at 16 weeks when the uterus becomes abdominal.

2. *Vaginal hysterectomy and repair* (i.e. including anterior colporrhaphy and posterior colpoperineorrhaphy) is usually the treatment of choice, especially if the woman has heavy periods or is post-menopausal. The uterosacral ligaments are plicated to prevent a subsequent enterocele. Sacrocolpopexy gives better results when there is also vault descent.

   Vaginal prolapse surgery involves a 3–6 day admission. Prophylaxis with broad-spectrum antibiotics reduces incidence of UTI (patient often catheterised) and infected vault haematoma. Thromboprophylaxis is wise. Secondary haemorrhage after 7–10 days may respond to antibiotics.

   A brown discharge occurs for 2–3 weeks afterwards, sometimes containing strands of suture material. Avoid heavy lifting for 2–3 months and intercourse is forbidden for 6 weeks. The vagina is slightly shortened but soon lengthens with regular intercourse.

3. Sacrospinous fixation: this is primarily a treatment to prevent or treat vaginal vault prolapse, and so is often combined with a vaginal hysterectomy. Using a specially designed instrument to allow placement of a suture through the sacrospinous ligament, the vaginal vault is elevated and suspended posteriorly. The major complications are bleeding (from large pelvic veins near the ligament) and buttock pain (which can last several months, but eventually settles without treatment).

4. An alternative operation is the *Manchester repair* (amputation of the cervix and suturing together of the transverse cervical ligaments). Subsequent pregnancy is still possible but cervical incompetence occurs and requires placement of a suture.

◆ Urinary incontinence

Distinguish:
– stress
– urgency
– continuous (fistula or congenital anomaly)

- overflow
- neurological causes
- infectious causes

Genuine stress incontinence

Troublesome involuntary leakage of urine when the intra-abdominal pressure is raised – e.g. on coughing, sneezing, laughing, running and lifting. It occurs to a slight degree in 10% of women who have had children, and is said to affect 50% of women at some time in their life at least once. The classic finding on examination is a cystocele and incontinence on coughing that can be prevented by digital paraurethral pressure (Bonney's test).

Stress incontinence can occur in the absence of these signs, however. Cystometry is normal apart from a low urethral closing pressure when the patient tries to squeeze the device.

The essential abnormality is descent of the upper urethra through the pelvic floor (levator ani) so that it is no longer compressed with the bladder when intra-abdominal pressure rises. Pubococcygeus (part of levator ani) is lax and no longer pulls the upper urethra forward, so that the posterior vesico-urethral angle is characteristically flat on a micturating cystogram (although this can be seen without any stress incontinence). The voluntary sphincter (the compressor urethrae, part of the deep perineal muscle) maintains continence at other times.

Making the correct *diagnosis:*
- symptoms may mislead (pad test), mixed picture always needs urodynamic assessment to clarify
- MSU always
- fluid charts/diary helps
- check drug history, ? diuretics

Treatment

Stress incontinence responds well to anatomical treatments (physiotherapy, surgery). Detrusor instability does not and may be exacerbated.

a) *Non-surgical. Pelvic floor exercises* – prolonged use essential. Physiotherapy or continence advice service helpful. The woman is taught how to elevate the perineum and 'contract the vagina', as if trying to prevent her bowels moving. This sensation can be demonstrated on examination by teaching her to pull up the perineum against the examining fingers or to squeeze the fingers or alternatively by one or two sessions of faradic stimulation by a physiotherapist.

If the woman is diligent with these exercises, they help in up to 75% of cases: they should be advised for all women after childbirth to prevent later stress incontinence.

A *ring pessary* may be inserted, and *practical measures* put in place for the elderly or infirm (check home arrangements). Incontinence pads can be provided by social services.

b) *Surgical.* A simple *anterior repair* (colporrhaphy) relieves symptoms in 70% in the short term. Long-term success is less. *Colposuspension* is much more effective, but a more major procedure. Long-term failures are less, but there is a 15% incidence of denovo detrusor instability following surgery. Because colposuspension is so effective at promoting continence some women are unable to empty their bladder adequately afterwards. Clean intermittent self-catheterisation is then useful (and preferred to being wet all the time). It exacerbates pre-existing instability (urgency) and should not be undertaken before full urodynamic assesment.

Following these operations a suprapubic catheter is needed for several days while normal voiding recovers. Elective section is usually advised for future pregnancies.

Sling procedures are effective but, invariably, erosion of the sling through the vaginal tissues is a future risk. A newer technique using a tension-free tape may not have this complication and may be the procedure of first choice in suitable women as it requires a very short hospital stay and the tape (inserted under local anaesthetic) is tightened only just sufficiently to prevent stress leakage when the patient coughs, so chronic retention and detrusor instability are rarely seen.

c) In the very elderly or infirm, transurethral injections of 'macro-plastique' at cystoscopy can be effective in reducing leakage, but often need to be repeated.

Urge incontinence

Urge incontinence means the sudden desire to void rapidly followed by incontinence. There is usually also frequency and nocturia. It is due to an 'irritable bladder' and is often difficult to treat. Cystometry shows detrusor contractions on minor pressure rises or even changes in posture. Assessment may include cytoscopy and IVU (stone or tumour), and UTI must be excluded.

Treatment

– bladder training and physiotherapy can help
drugs are some help in 50%: all contraindicated with significant degrees of outflow obstruction:
oxybutynin: reduces detrusor contractions. Anticholinergic side-effects, especially dry mouth, constipation, blurred vision, tachycardia. Unwise in the elderly
imipramine: at night, can help nocturia
tolterodine: Detrusitol 1–2 mg b.d., antimuscarinic, good for urgency and frequency. Review treatment need after 6-month course.

Bladder instillations or hydrostatic dilatation under epidural can be tried in resistant cases, but long-term effectiveness poor.

Long-term detrusor instability is disabling. Support groups can offer useful advice.

Continuous dribbling

Occurs with:
– vesicovaginal fistula (radiotherapy, carcinoma or prolonged obstructed labour)
– retention with overflow, when the bladder will be palpable. This is usually due to diabetic neuropathy

Note: Remember common and rare causes of incontinence:
– pregnancy: frequently get stress incontinence and nocturia ± UTI
– multiple sclerosis

61

- cord compression
- pelvic tumours
- fistula (malignancy, radiotherapy, trauma)
- diabetes

◆ Gynaecological backache

Most backache is *not* gynaecological in origin.

Gynaecological backache is continuous, bilateral aching, below the iliac crests, quite unlike lumbar root pain (sudden onset, worse on movement, radiation, tenderness). Relevant gynaecological clues are cyclical pain, dyspareunia, malignancy, UTI.

Consider:
- uterovaginal prolapse
- endometriosis
- chronic salpingitis
- carcinoma of the cervix
- vertebral metastases

Straight leg raising and sensory testing of lower limbs may be indicated. X-ray of lumbar spine is rarely helpful unless metastases are suspected.

Retroversion of the uterus is common (15% population) and rarely causes backache. A Hodge pessary can be inserted to hold the uterus anteverted for a few weeks. If this relieves the symptoms then ventrosuspension (suturing the round ligaments to the rectus sheath) may be justified and can be performed at laparoscopy.

In endometriosis and chronic salpingitis the pain tends to be worse before periods and there will be other symptoms (dyspareunia, menorrhagia and discharge). Laparoscopy is indicated.

◆ Breast examination

Many carcinomas still present as large lumps, and teaching *self-examination* of the breast is probably a useful method of screening, e.g. using the following method:
1. The best time to feel for lumps routinely is after a period, when lumpiness (fibroadenosis) is commonly felt.
2. Look at the breasts in the mirror, then raise the arms, looking for asymmetry or nipple inversion.
3. Use the flat of the hand and four fingers to feel for lumps (the fingertips detect the normal lumpiness of the glandular tissue).
4. Feel *all* the breast (with the opposite hand) systematically ('like the face of a clock'), pressing the breast against the ribs. Explain how the axillary tail of the breast tissue extends into the armpit and should not be missed.

A *mammogram* is a soft-tissue X-ray that enhances masses due to the inherent contrast properties of breast tissue on X-ray. They tend to be easier to interpret after the menopause as there are fewer cyclical changes occurring. A routine screening programme has been set up in the UK offering mammography to the over 50s. The test can be uncomfortable or even painful, but will detect lumps over 0.5 cm with good accuracy. Irregularity suggests carcinoma but *all* masses should be referred for surgical review.

Outpatient clinic procedures using fine needle aspiration (FNA) with immediately available cytology results have reduced the need for surgical removal of lumps and provide rapid reassurance to many women.

Breast lumps
- fibroadenoma
- fibroadenosis
- cyst
- carcinoma

1. A *fibroadenoma* (age 20–30) is a lump that is characteristically very mobile ('the breast mouse'). It is treated by excision biopsy – 'no woman should have a lump in the breast'.
2. *Fibroadenosis* (age 20–50) is due to multiple small cysts (epitheliosis blocking the ducts), usually in the upper outer quadrant. It is uncomfortable and tender and is worse before a period, settling down once the period is established. It tends to be worse when periods are irregular and there may be other features of premenstrual tension (fluid retention, headache, irritability). It is cured during a pregnancy. Management involves:
   - reassure and see in 2 weeks when it will have settled
   - mild analgesics and a firm bra. Frusemide 40 mg daily for the 4 days before a period often helps. Alternatively, bromocriptine or danazol are both effective
   - if further reassurance is needed, aspiration of one of the larger cysts or mammography (shows multiple rounded lesions of variable density) can be helpful
3. A *cyst* (age 40–50) usually appears suddenly, often just after a period and most commonly in the last 5 years before the menopause. It may be in an area of fibroadenosis (the pathology is the same). Treatment is by aspiration and biopsy is unnecessary, provided:
   - the lump disappears completely
   - the fluid is not uniformly bloodstained
   - the fluid is negative on cytology
   - the cyst does not rapidly reform (see in 1 month)
   Cysts *never* occur after 1 year postmenopause.
4. *Carcinoma* of the breast (most common age 40–80). Over the age of 60 a lump will be a carcinoma (unless there is a clear history of recent severe bruising, when it may be fat necrosis). The lump is single, hard, irregular and non-tender and there may be tethering or nipple inversion or discharge, skin nodules or palpable nodes.

   Prognosis depends on whether metastases are already present (25% even in patients with early lesions) and not on the method of removing the primary. Simple lumpectomy followed by radiotherapy produces as good a survival rate as any other method.

   Adjuvant therapy now makes radical mastectomy an infrequent operation, which is good because the outcome is the same with lump excision and drugs/radiotherapy and the rate of complications (emotional and physical) of radical surgery is high.

2. Sexually transmitted disease

- HIV
- syphilis
- gonorrhoea
- NSU (non-specific urethritis)
- genital herpes
- genital warts
- molluscum contagiosum
- pediculosis pubis
- tropical (chancroid, LGV)

Scabies, *Candida* and trichomoniasis can also be spread by sexual contact. Hepatitis B, *Giardia*, *Shigella* and amoebiasis are probably transmissible by the venereal route.

Some of these infections carry particular risks in pregnancy.

There are *two important principles* in the management of all sexually transmitted diseases:

1. If one infection is present, always exclude the others.
2. Trace and treat all contacts, a difficult task best performed by specially trained nurses or social workers.

◆ HIV infection and AIDS

Acquired immune deficiency syndrome was first described in homosexual men in the USA in 1981: presentations with *Pneumocystis carinii* pneumonia, mucosal candidiasis and Kaposi's sarcoma suggested an immune deficiency. Retrospective searches indicated that cases had probably also been occurring in the 1970s.

Infection with human immunodeficiency virus (HIV) is now recognised as affecting both sexes, homosexual and heterosexual, and can be passed from mother to infant. *Transmission* is predominantly by sexual contact but can be by administration of blood products (haemophiliacs), by the use of contaminated needles (intravenous drug abusers), via other body fluids, or may be vertical.

The *risk of transmission* of HIV is increased when the *carrier* has/is:

- high degree of immunosuppression
- low CD4 lymphocyte count
- in the later stages of HIV infection or has AIDS

and when the *recipient* has/is:

- genital tract infection, inflammation, ulceration or trauma
- an IUD in situ
- not protected by a condom
- allowing anal sexual contact (mucosal abrasion)

Epidemiology

Worldwide:
- there are > 33 million people infected with HIV (1998)
- > 1500 children are newly infected every day
- new infection is commonest in SE Asia, Southern and Central Africa
- heterosexual spread is a big problem (a third of cases now occur in women)

In the UK (at the end of 1998):
- over 5500 women were HIV-positive
- 10% of HIV positives are in the > 50 year age group
- nearly 2000 had developed AIDS
- diagnosis may only be made because/after a child is diagnosed
- reported cases are always an underestimate of the total
- HIV occurs in all health districts, but Greater London, Edinburgh and Dundee report the highest prevalence
- the majority (> 85%) of HIV and AIDS in children is due to transmission from mother to child before/during birth and by breast-feeding
- in London 1 in 500 births are to HIV-positive mothers

(See also Chapter 4 *Obstetrics*.)

Pathogenesis of HIV infection

Most HIV carriers are asymptomatic; some will develop malignancies or opportunistic infections.

Following new infection with HIV, over 50% of individuals develop symptoms within 2–6 weeks: fever, arthralgia, myalgia, headaches, rash, lymphadenopathy, diarrhoea (and are viraemic at this time). The immune response and seroconversion to HIV-positive takes up to 12 weeks, sometimes much longer. Once positive, they can pass on the virus for many years. The infection then has a latent, asymptomatic, phase of 10 or more years (see Fig. 4). During this phase, gradual immunosuppression (evidenced by falling CD4 counts and defective T cell function) occurs.

HIV selectively infects T cells, macrophages and other lymphocytes with the CD4 antigen after which its DNA is incorporated into

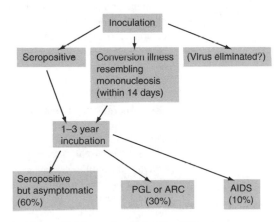

Fig. 4 Natural history of events after HIV exposure

the host cell's genome. If the cell is activated, e.g. by another viral antigen, the HIV-infected cell is killed as a result, thereby decreasing the immune defences of the patient. The human immunodeficiency virus can also infect some tissues directly, e.g. the CNS, leading to neurological features.

The immunosuppression presents finally as the disease AIDS. There are many presentations, often with unusual or rare malignancies or opportunistic infections (e.g. *Candida, Pneumocystis*).

Clinical aspects of AIDS

The clinical picture can include:
- weight loss, fever, lymphadenopathy
- dry cough (*Pneumocystis*)
- persistent oral thrush
- purple skin lesions (Kaposi's sarcoma)
- diarrhoea (*Salmonella*, CMV, *Cryptosporidium*)
- perianal ulceration (herpes simplex)
- headaches (cerebral abscess)
- progressive dementia (HIV encephalopathy)
- cachexia and death

1. 50% present with *Pneumocystis* infection, with dry cough and fever but often no signs and a normal CXR initially. There is hypoxia and a marked reduction in carbon monoxide transfer. Bronchoscopy is essential for diagnosis (midzone brushings). Asthma tends to worsen. Treatment is with high-dose *Septrin 9* (480 mg) *tabs b.d.* 80% get a maculopapular rash on Septrin, which is not an indication to stop treatment but if the rash involves mucosae treatment is changed to pentamidine. *Candida* pneumonitis and atypical TB also occur.

2. *Oral thrush* can be extremely difficult to eradicate, and commonly involves the oesophagus. Long-term ketoconazole (Nizoral) is needed. Leukoplakia also occurs in the mouth and can be mistaken for thrush.

3. *Kaposi's sarcoma* is a vascular neoplasm previously seen as an indolent condition in elderly males. Kaposi's plaques typically appear first on the palate. Purple skin lesions resembling bruises enlarge into nodules. Gut involvement occurs. The prognosis is better with Kaposi's alone, without opportunistic infections. There is also an increased incidence of B cell lymphoma.

4. *Diarrhoea* is a common problem due to *Salmonella*, CMV (can cause toxic dilatation of the colon), and *Cryptosporidium*. Cryptosporidiosis causes profuse watery diarrhoea (like cholera) and is diagnosed using a Ziehl-Neelsen stain. It is rapidly fatal. There were only 12 cases in the world literature before 1982. There is often an associated bacteraemia (e.g. salmonellosis) which is difficult to eradicate with antibiotics.

5. *Perianal ulceration* and induration occurs due to chronic herpes simplex infection. It responds well to acyclovir. Squamous carcinoma of the anal margin is more common (possibly associated with wart virus).

66

6. 20% present with *CNS symptoms*. Encephalitis can occur due to CMV, herpes simplex or *Cryptococcus*. CT scan is indicated to exclude a cerebral abscess (toxoplasmosis or *Candida*) and lumbar puncture may be indicated. Brain biopsy worsens prognosis.

CMV retinitis can cause bilateral blindness. Cotton wool spots on the retina are highly suggestive of impending opportunistic infection.

Cerebral atrophy and dementia can occur, thought to be due to direct invasion with HIV. *Dementia* is a possibility even in those successfully treated for opportunistic infections.

7. *Death* occurs 1–2 years after diagnosis. Survival depends on presenting disease. Infections become more frequent and more difficult to eradicate. Weight loss and wasting occur even in the absence of infections. In addition to infections, presenile dementia can occur due to primary brain infection with HIV.

Testing for HIV   Two scenarios exist:

1. 'Voluntary named testing' – patient and carers (only if the patient agrees) know the result. Knowing the HIV status allows follow-up, advice on reducing transmission to sexual partners, and early treatment if appropriate (antenatal testing falls into this group).

2. 'Voluntary (unlinked) anonymous testing' – test result unknown on an individual basis either to patient or carer. This strategy was useful for collection of epidemiological data. Unlinked testing using samples taken for other purposes can be done without specific consent but the patient may withhold permission if they are aware that such programmes are being undertaken.

Counselling before and after the results are known is vital.

Advantages of testing:
– epidemiological data may aid prevention programmes
– treatment of infected individuals is most successful if begun early. This is especially true when trying to reduce mother-to-baby transmission
– may influence decisions on sexual practice, having a family, etc.
– allows alteration of management of an infected pregnant woman to lessen risk of transmission to fetus
– allows carers to reduce risk of infection to themselves. (**Note**: At the moment, carers cannot insist that a patient be tested, unless the patient is not in a fit state to make that decision)

Disadvantages of testing:
– psychological factors enormously important. May enhance risk-taking behaviour (drugs, unsafe sexual practices may seem acceptable). May lead to collapse of coping strategy with acute psychiatric effects
– may restrict access to medical care and tests if carer wrongly perceives excess risk, e.g. to staff
– social, financial and insurance consequences

Laboratory tests   HIV antibody testing initially. Detection of viral antigens in cells (by immunofluorescence or Western blot immunoelectrophoresis) confirms infection. Detection of antibodies confirms persisting infection but not all carriers develop the same antibody response (Fig. 5).

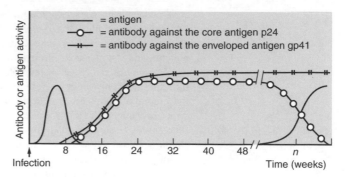

Fig. 5 Development of antibody response to HIV

Pre-test counselling
- consider *informed* consent and education as priorities
- discuss other sexually transmitted diseases, 'safe' sex and contraception
- explain HIV and AIDS and their interrelationship
- explain modes of transmission
- discuss the advantages of knowing your HIV status, especially to pregnant women
- explain how the result will come through and who will know. Discuss the follow-up plans should the test be positive
- reassure about confidentiality

Confirming the presence of HIV antibodies is a life-changing event. The information is sometimes a shock and the patient needs to express fears, discuss uncertainties and come to terms with changes in lifestyle.

Contraception and HIV
- condoms reduce the risk of transmission to partners. Other forms of contraception with higher safety may be used in addition to avoid pregnancy
- diaphragms do not offer protection, the female condom (Femshield or Femidom) *may*
- nonoxinol '9' may be useful in its own right to lessen transmission
- combined oral contraceptive depresses the immune system but there is no evidence that it worsens outlook in HIV carriers. Its effectiveness makes it ideal for use with a condom
- injectables are safe and avoid compliance problems, e.g. in drug abusers
- IUD should be avoided as it may enhance transmission due to intercurrent PID or trauma at insertion
- sterilisation carries surgical hazard but is otherwise safe
- postcoital contraception (but not with IUD) is safe

Several useful booklets are available on HIV, AIDS and HIV testing (see p. 74).

◆ Syphilis

There remain a substantial number of cases of syphilis per year in the UK: over 1000 are notified annually. It is caused by the spirochaete

Treponema pallidum which can invade intact mucosa or enter through abrasions anywhere on the skin.

The four stages are:

1. The *primary chancre* develops about 3 weeks (9–90 days) after contact, usually on the vulva or penis (or anus in homosexuals, resembling a fissure).

   A pink papule breaks into an ulcer which is painless, rounded and oozes serum. Untreated, it heals in 3–8 weeks. The inguinal nodes are usually enlarged, but are rubbery and non-tender.

   Diagnosis involves dark-ground illumination of the ulcer fluid for spirochaetes: may need repeating daily to confirm. Serology does not become positive until around 6 weeks – repeat monthly for 3 months. Keep the ulcer clean with saline but never give antibiotics until the diagnosis is certain. Follow up for 2 years.

2. *Secondary syphilis* develops about 6 weeks after the chancre appears, with fever, myalgia, malaise and:
   - rash (non-itchy, symmetrical, maculopapular lesions involving palms and soles; sometimes alopecia) – 75%
   - generalised lymphadenopathy (rubbery and non-tender and including epitrochlear and suboccipital nodes) – 50%
   - mucosal ulcers (snail track) – 10%, or perineal 'warts' (condylomata lata) – 10%. Both teem with spirochaetes if dark-ground illumination is used on the serum

   Untreated, these manifestations resolve over a period of months and the patient passes into the stage of *latent syphilis* with positive serology but no other involvement, including aortic (CXR) and CSF (lumbar puncture). Even without treatment 60% experience no further progression.

3. *Tertiary syphilis* is rarely seen nowadays. It occurs 3–10 years after primary infection and is characterised by gummas (granulomas), mainly of skin, mucosa and bone (and rarely viscera) which heal with penicillin treatment.

4. *Cardiovascular* or *neurological complications* develop in about 10% of untreated cases after 5–30 years. They are due to endarteritis and fibrotic damage to the aortic ring:
   - aortic incompetence
   - angina
   - aortic aneurysm (ascending and calcified)

   and to damage to the meninges and nerve roots:
   - meningovascular syphilis (headache, cranial nerve palsies, root pain)
   - tabes dorsalis (dorsal column degeneration)
   - GPI (cortical degeneration and dementia)

Serology Current screening tests for syphilis are the VDRL (introduced after the Second World War) the TPHA and the FTA.

1. The *VDRL* detects an antibody (reagin) which is present in high titre in syphilis and causes clumping of lipoidal antigens (flocculation).

   It is positive in 75% of primary syphilis cases and is ideal for follow-up because it becomes negative with treatment.

False positives occur in:
- viral illness, vaccinations
- glandular fever
- SLE
- rheumatoid arthritis

2. The *TPHA* (introduced in 1967) detects specific anti-treponemal antibodies that haemagglutinate sheep red cells. False positives are less likely.

   If only one test is positive repeat the screen; if both tests are positive perform an FTA.

3. The *FTA* (introduced 1964) was devised to overcome the problem of false positives. It labels the treponemes with specific fluorescent antibodies. It is the most sensitive test and is highly specific. It is the first to become positive (at 6 weeks) and remains positive for life. It is time-consuming and expensive.

Management

1. In pregnancy all women are screened once at booking. Screening can be repeated if the woman is considered to be at risk, at 34 weeks.

2. Syphilis confirmed by FTA is treated with procaine penicillin 900 mg daily by i.m. injection for at least 10 days. In patients with penicillin allergy, oral erythromycin for 2 weeks is an alternative.

   Inadequate treatment leaves the patient susceptible to the late complications. Treatment even late in pregnancy usually leads to the birth of a healthy child.

3. Untreated syphilis in pregnancy tends to cause abortion or stillbirth. Later pregnancies in a syphilitic woman can run to term and the child may have *congenital syphilis* (bloodborne, therefore no primary stage), with:
   - rash and lymphadenopathy
   - bloodstained nasal discharge (osteochondritis)
   - gummas and neurosyphilis (late)

Diagnosis in a baby is proved by the IgM-FTA test, although this may not be positive until 9 weeks. It is treated with penicillin.

◆ Gonorrhoea

There were 50 000 new cases/year in the 1960s and 1970s, falling to < 12 000 by 1994. However, recently the numbers have risen again – especially among young females (16–24 years) and in men of all ages. In 1996 the incidence was 44 cases/100 000 population. The incidence due to homosexual contact appears to have increased as well.

Neisseria gonorrhoeae is a Gram-negative intracellular diplococcus that invades tissue not covered with stratified squamous epithelium (urethra, cervix, Bartholin's glands). Trichomoniasis coexists in 60%.

In men, it causes dysuria and purulent urethral discharge 3–9 days after contact, but in 20% it is mild and unrecognised. In women, it is often symptomless but about 40% develop symptoms such as dysuria, frequency and vaginal discharge about 2 weeks after contact. It can persist as a chronic and contagious disease for years and is the commonest cause of 'blocked tubes'.

Diagnosis: take charcoal swabs from the urethra, endocervix, rectum and (?) pharynx. Transport promptly to the lab in Stuart's medium. In men, a Gram stain of discharge is 95% accurate, but in women commensal organisms complicate the picture and culture is necessary. Amplification techniques with PCR (polymerase chain reactions) allow rapid accurate diagnosis.

Complications
- acute salpingitis, irregular menses, pelvic pain
- bartholinitis (epididymitis men)
- anorectal infection occurs in up to 50% of women and in homosexual men (anal sex)
- pharyngitis (oral sex)
- vulvovaginitis (children)
- bacteraemia (fever, rash, septic arthritis)
- neonatal ophthalmitis (blinding)

Gonorrhoea must always be suspected in acute salpingitis (20% risk if gonococcus is untreated) especially if there has been no recent delivery or abortion and the woman does not have an IUD.

Treatment
Best as a single dose – compliance is excellent and contact treatment is more likely to succeed. Use any of:
- i.m. ceftriaxone 250 mg
- oral ciprofloxacin 500 mg
- oral ofloxacin 400 mg
- oral azithromycin 2 g

Resistance is emerging to amoxicillin + probenecid – no longer favoured.

In pregnancy use ceftriaxone or spectinomycin.

Always refer to STD clinic. Follow-up is essential, with contact tracing and screening for other STD.

Gonococcal vaccine may be available in the future.

◆ Chlamydia

Chlamydia trachomatis infection is usually asymptomatic in women but non-specific discharge and dysuria may occur. 10% of carriers develop serious tubal disease and chlamydia is therefore a major cause of infertility (see Chapter 1). Chlamydia causes acute PID more commonly than gonococcus. In severe cases, perihepatic inflammation occurs with upper abdominal signs and symptoms (Fitz-Hugh-Curtis syndrome). Reiter's syndrome is a triad of chlamydial arthritis, conjunctivitis and mucosal ulceration.

In males it can cause urethritis and discharge, and epididymitis.

In neonates, conjunctivitis ('sticky eye') occurs 5 days to 2 weeks after birth.

The cervix often looks normal. Diagnosis is by antigen detection and requires special endocervical samples, put into a tissue culture medium. Because of delay or because inappropriate swabs were taken, the diagnosis often used to be missed.

Treatment
Use oral doxycycline 200 mg followed by 100 mg daily for 7 days (erythromycin if pregnant). Single dose azithromycin 1 g is an

alternative (but more expensive). Repeat swabs after 2 and 4 weeks to ensure negative.

Coexistent anaerobic infection requires metronidazole.

Contact tracing is important and treatment is necessary.

Note: remember that the patient may be pregnant.

◆ Non-specific urethritis

NSU is now the commonest reason for male referral to GU medicine clinics and although treatment is straightforward, referral is helpful to take advantage of the contact-tracing schemes and screening for other STDs. There are over 100 000 cases of NSU (male and female) notified annually. In men, chlamydia accounts for about 50%; the other organisms remain uncertain but mycoplasma and *Ureaplasma* are suspected.

Men develop dysuria and mucoid urethral discharge, usually 2–3 weeks after contact. It can be assumed to be due to *Chlamydia* species. Make the diagnosis on a Gram-stain of the discharge – shows pus cells but no gonococci. *Complications* are prostatitis, epididymitis and Reiter's syndrome – if chlamydia (5% overall). Treatment: 10 days of doxycycline 100 mg orally. It tends to recur and can be very difficult to eradicate.

◆ Genital herpes

This is the commonest cause of vulvovaginitis ulceration in the UK. It is due to herpes simplex virus (type 2 > type 1). Infection may be primary, recurrent, atypical or asymptomatic. The clustering of vesicles is very distinctive, but syphilis must always be excluded in any genital ulceration. Definitive diagnosis is by swabs and cervical scrapings for viral culture (which produces characteristic cell changes). Single serology tests are largely unhelpful (but will be positive after oral infection or 'cold sores'). Oro-genital sex can transmit HSV. Non-sexual transmission has never been reported. Paired sera will show a rising titre after a primary attack.

The first attack: about 5 days after contact a burning sensation develops, then a cluster of tiny vesicles appears which soon rupture, leaving painful erosions, usually on the vulva but sometimes on the cervix. The primary infection is often severe, with fever and malaise, nerve root involvement (pain, difficulty micturating) and painful inguinal lymphadenopathy or iliac fossa pain (the cervix drains to the iliac nodes). Rarely, meningitis or hepatitis may be seen. Cervical herpes usually causes severe necrotic ulceration, but the virus can be shed from a normal-looking cervix.

The patient may be unable to pass urine: try local anaesthetic gel or catheterisation (may need to be suprapubic) in the most severe cases. If on the pill, skip the next period by running two O/C packets together as pads will be uncomfortable and tampons out of the question. Avoid sexual contact. Antiviral therapy (oral acyclovir) may be started on suspicion of herpes – do not wait for confirmation. Topical aciclovir is ineffective. Early treatment curtails the duration of symptoms but does not prevent latency developing. Secondary bacterial or fungal infection should be treated.

Viral shedding continues even when asymptomatic – 70% of transmission to partners occurred *between* clinical attacks in one study. The *risk of viral transmission to others* is greater:
– in the first 12 months after the initial attack
– during a symptomatic episiode
– in people with frequent recurrent attacks
– with type 2 HSV infection

Recurrent attacks are less severe and are usually precipitated by sexual intercourse. Suppressive therapy reduces the frequency and severity of attacks – continuous therapy for 6–12 months if >8 attacks/year?

Notes on treatment
– the ulcers will heal in 10 days as long as secondary infection is prevented. Potassium permanganate baths are soothing and povidone-iodine helps prevent secondary infection
– analgesics are needed if root pain develops. Urinary hesitancy always resolves: *urethral* catheterisation should be avoided if possible
– if secondary infection occurs use Septrin, which does not mask syphilis (check serology at 3 months to exclude syphilis)
– genital herpes in the last month of pregnancy is an indication for elective section (neonatal encephalitis can occur)
– aciclovir is a potent and specific antiviral agent, which is active against herpes simplex types 1 and 2: the pain and other symptoms of the primary infection are reduced and subsequent recurrence rate may be reduced. Aciclovir cream only reduces the severity of recurrent episodes if applied early (before vesicles appear). Continuous use has been shown to suppress recurrent attacks, but when treatment stops recurrences return. It has no serious side-effects. Valaciclovir and famciclovir are newer alternatives to acyclovir
– severe cases require hospitalisation if there is retention of urine or chest complications with pneumonia-like symptoms
– herpes can be life-threatening in immunosuppressed patients

◆ Genital warts (condylomata accuminata)

Caused by HPV and transmitted sexually. The incubation period is around 3 months (1–6 months). Although most carriers have no visible warts, they are still infectious to others. Most genital warts occur on the vulva and perineum, but may extend up the vagina. They can become large, particularly in immunosuppressed patients. They are unsightly, cause itching, irritation and discharge and they may bleed. In a few patients, treatment is ineffective but, like warts on the hand, they will eventually disappear. 25% have another STD as well – check.

Management
1. Inspect the cervix for lesions (reported association with CIN). Take a smear.
2. Topical podophyllin (10–25%) in spirit or in tincture of benzoin: applied weekly to the warts and washed off 6 hours later. It is very irritant to normal skin, which should be protected during application with Vaseline. If skin irritation occurs, 2% hydrocortisone

cream is useful. Some podophyllin is absorbed and as it is teratogenic it must never be used in pregnancy. The consort should be treated if warts are present or should use a sheath to prevent infection.

3. Multiple warts are best treated by diathermy under general anaesthetic. Laser is very useful (preferred over diathermy) with less residual scarring.

4. Exclude other venereal infections. Trichomoniasis commonly coexists.

Molluscum contagiosum causes painless, fleshy papules that are easily recognised because of a central umbilification, out of which cheesy material can be squeezed. They are caused by a very large DNA pox virus. They are spread by direct contact and can occur on any part of the body. Podophyllin is effective.

◆ Pubic lice (pediculosis pubis)

Infestation often presents with intense pruritus and dermatitis from scratching, about 1 month after contact. Confirm the diagnosis by identifying nits (hand lens useful) attached to the pubic hair shafts, or adult crabs. Treatment is with topical malathion ('Derbac') or phenothrin ('Full Marks') in cream or lotion form which is washed off after 8 hours – treat the whole body.

◆ Tropical venereal infections

- chancroid
- lymphogranuloma venereum
- granuloma inguinale

1. *Chancroid*: important as it can mimic primary syphilis. It is largely confined to seaports of the Far East, Africa and South America. There are very few cases annually in the UK, most occurring in foreign travellers.

    1–14 days after contact, multiple painful ulcers develop on the genitals. Inguinal nodes become tender and enlarge and can develop into an abscess. Diagnosis usually has to be clinical but syphilis (usually presenting with a single painful ulcer with rubbery non-tender nodes) must be excluded by dark-ground illumination. Organism is *Haemophilus ducreyi* which is extremely difficult to culture. Can be treated with co-amoxiclav or erythromycin for 7 days or with a single dose of azithromycin. Co-trimoxazole has the advantage that it does not mask syphilis.

2. *Lymphogranuloma venereum (LGV):* About 1–3 weeks after contact, small painless ulcers develop which usually go unnoticed as they heal quickly in women. Initial ulceration causes diagnostic confusion with other ulcerative lesions of the vulva. The second phase of the disease causes chronic inguinal lymphadenitis, often weeks later, usually with fever and weight loss. Finally, after months or years, untreated individuals develop necrotic lymph nodes with chronic sinus formation and caseous discharge, labial perforations, fibrotic scarring with fistulae, rectal and urethral

strictures and lymphoedema. Epitheliomas can develop in the involved skin.

Caused by specific serotypes of chlamydia and is most common in tropical coastal areas. Immunofluorescence tests help in diagnosis as chlamydia culture can be difficult. Treat with doxycycline for 14 days.

3. *Granuloma inguinale* is an uncommon chronic skin condition virtually confined to coloured races in tropical regions. Incubation is around 6 weeks (often much less) but can be as long as 3 months. Non-tender nodules appear and may coalesce. Painless ulcers with a deep red base develop, with ulcerating granulomas, in the perineal or inguinal region, eventually healing with fibrosis. Diagnosis is made on biopsy. It has been diagnosed in the endometrium and parametrium on surgical specimens. The causative agent is Calymmatobacterium granulomatis. Treat with tetracyclines.

◆ AIDS resources

1. Avert (Aids Education and Research Trust) Produces several useful booklets on AIDS.
   Tel.   01403 210202
   Website   http://www.avert.org/
   E-mail   http://www.avert@dial.pipex.com
2. The Terrence Higgins Trust has produced:
   – Women with HIV and AIDS
   – HIV, AIDS and Pregnancy
   – HIV Testing
   Tel. Helpline   020 7242 1010
   Website   http://www.tht.org.uk
3. The BMA Foundation for AIDS has published:
   – Take the HIV Test
   Tel.   020 7388 2544
   Website   http://www.bmaids.demon.co.uk/

3. Family planning

The world's population is currently just over 6 billion, an increase of over 1 billion since the third edition of this book was written! Birth rates are steady – even dropping – in most Western countries but continue to escalate rapidly in the underdeveloped world. Family planning presents both personal and global issues of urgency.

The *ideal contraceptive* does not exist. If it did, it would (be):
– 100% effective and reversible
– 100% safe, without undesirable side-effects
– independent of intercourse
– not require high motivation to use reliably
– effective pre-fertilisation, which increases acceptability
– independent of medical advice
– cheap
– have other beneficial effects (prevention of STD or reduction of gynaecological cancer)
– probably be best under female control (since she is the one who gets pregnant)

◆ Effectiveness

– depends on reliability of use of the method
– can be enhanced by correct explanation by health care professional
– usually calculated/expressed as failure rate/100 woman years (i.e. 100 women using method correctly over 1 year, or 1 woman over 100 years)

$$\text{Failure rate} = \frac{\text{Total accidental pregnancies}}{\text{Total months of exposure}} \times 1200$$

– failure rates (Table 2) lowest for long-term users (who find method acceptable) and for older women (reduced fertility)
– method very variable in different age (Table 3) and ethnic groups

Table 2 Examples of failure rates (Oxford FPA Study, *Lancet* 1982) (expressed as rate/100 woman years)

	Women 25–34 years	Women > 35 years
Sterilisation		
Male	0.08	0.08
Female	0.45	0.08
Combined O/C	0.38	0.23
POP	2.5	0.5
IUD	(surveys other than Oxford FPA suggest 0.5–1.0 for modern Cu-based coils)	
Diaphragm	5.5	2.8
Condom (male)	6.0	2.9

Table 3 Current usage of contraceptive methods (Great Britain) (General Household Survey, 1991 (OPCS 1992))

Main method	Overall	18–19 years	20–24 years	30–34 years	>40 years
Sterilisation (male or female)	25%	0%	1%	21%	50%
Pill (comb. or POP)	23%	46%	48%	25%	4%
Condom	16%	15%	14%	17%	13%
IUD	5%				
Pregnant/trying to conceive	16%				
No partner	16%				

◆ General advice

- counselling requires accurate transfer of information, leaving the woman/couple to decide for themselves which method to choose
- contraception (all methods) is *less* risky than pregnancy (Table 4)
- cultural and social factors may dictate the couple's choice of options
- non-contraceptive benefits (STD, ovarian cancer protection) may influence choice
- accurate past medical history is essential (thrombosis, hypertension, pelvic sepsis)
- family planning discussions are a good opportunity to raise other issues, e.g. smears/breast examination/sex education/STD
- prolonged lactation significantly reduces fertility and could greatly enhance family planning prospects, particularly for Third World countries. In the UK it permits the use of 'less reliable' methods with greater confidence, but remember to discuss change in method when breastfeeding is discontinued

Table 4 Death rates/100 000 users of contraception

	<35 years	>35 years
O/C pill		
Non-smokers	2	12
Smokers	8	40
IUD	1	1
TOP	2	3
Pregnancy	15	20

◆ The combined pill

Has been available since the 1960s but new formulations are appearing regularly, usually with a lower oestrogen content and safer progestogens. Oestrogen content varies between 20 μg and 50 μg. The lowest dose that provides good cycle control and fewest side-effects is recommended. An RCGP survey in 1986 reported that 95% of sexually active women <30 years of age had used a combined O/C at some time.

Action: the combined oral contraceptive prevents ovulation by inhibiting follicular maturation and blocking positive feedback by oestrogen, thus eliminating the LH surge.
- reduces ability of cervical mucus to allow sperm passage
- changes endometrium to make it less favourable towards blastocyst implantation

Formulations:
- continuous doses of oestrogen and progestogens
- phasic (variable doses)
- formulations including dummy tablets, allowing continuous 28-day usage (known as everyday or 'ED' formulations – unpopular in UK, but widely used in Europe)

The withdrawal bleed is the endometrial response to cessation of administered hormones, not a true menstrual bleed. Follicular activity returns during the pill-free interval: missing pills at the beginning or end of the packet is more likely to result in unwanted ovulation than if pills are missed mid-packet.

The '7 day rule' (FPA) is useful: it takes 7 daily pills to reliably suppress ovarian function. If pills are missed, extra contraception is required for the next 7 days, and the pill-free interval should be omitted by running two packets together if <7 pills remain in the packet from which pills are missed.

Minor side-effects are rare but include:
- fluid retention, breast tenderness, nausea, vaginal discharge (?oestrogenic)
- acne, hirsutism, weight gain, loss of libido, dry vagina, depression (?progestogen component)

Serious side-effects/risks

1. *Venous thromboembolism*. Change in clotting factors: reduced antithrombin III, enhanced platelet aggregation and elevated fibrinogen predispose to venous thrombosis. Fibrinolysis is also enhanced (which is protective) but *not* in smokers, hence smokers are at far greater risk.
   - the risk of venous thromboembolism in healthy women not taking an oral contraceptive is about 5/100 000/year
   - combined O/C with second-generation progestogens; risk is 15/100 000/year
   - combined O/C with third-generation progestogens; risk is 25/100 000/year
   - in pregnancy the risk is 60/100 000 pregnancies
   Clotting returns to normal within 4–8 weeks of stopping the pill. *In healthy women the combined O/C need not be discontinued prior to uncomplicated laparoscopic sterilisation.* Risk does not increase with increasing duration of use. Smoking habits, immobility (e.g. RTA, major surgery) and the *dose* of oestrogen are more significant than duration of use.

2. *Arterial disease*. Most users show small but significant rises in systolic and diastolic BP. Lower doses of either oestrogen or progestogen reduce the effect. Risk of myocardial infarction and CVA are related to concurrent hypertension. Third-generation progestogens (gestodene, desogestrel) have fewer adverse effects on lipids than first- or second-generation alternatives (norethisterone, levonorgestrel) – but have greater venous thromboembolic risks (see above).

Regular BP reviews are essential in O/C users. Smoking plus hypertension carries the highest risk. Excess risk of myocardial infarction in smokers taking the combined O/C is 21 × controls.

Over the age of 35, non-smokers may continue the O/C until age 50, depending on other risk factors. *Smokers should stop at age 35.*

3. *Malignancy*. Carcinoma of endometrium and ovary are *less* common in combined O/C users. Other cancers may be more common but as yet no *causative* links have been proven.

Endometrial cancer is reduced by 50% in 'ever-users' (protection greater with longer use). *Ovarian cancer* is reduced overall by 40% (protection lasts for around 15 years after stopping O/C).

Breast cancer. Data are conflicting. Lower oestrogen doses probably present lower risks. The increase in risk probably applies to women taking the O/C early (before their first pregnancy) and over a long period. The UK National Case Control Study (1989) suggests an excess of early-pill-users in women diagnosed with cancer of the breast below age 36. Vessey (1989) suggested that use in women >25 years carried little or no increased risk. In summary, the risk of breast cancer is approx. 2:1000 in women under 36. The combined O/C increases this risk by a further 1:1000 (the 'excess' risk). The lifetime incidence of breast cancer in women is 1:11 (although many die from other causes). The risks of breast cancer in older pill-users are unclear and no accurate data agree as yet.

Women with a strong family history of breast cancer *probably* do not increase their risk of the disease by taking the O/C. (They may choose other methods 'in case'.) If they wish to start the O/C, advise the lowest possible oestrogen dose for the shortest time and increase surveillance. Choice of progestogen may be important but the evidence is conflicting. The POP may be preferable.

Cancer of the cervix: Sexual activity clouds the issue. Smoking also increases the risk. The association between cancer of the cervix and O/C use may be causal or casual. The Oxford FPA Study (1983) suggested increased risk with prolonged duration of use. 3-yearly smears are recommended but sexual lifestyle (multiple partners, coincident STD) may indicate more frequent assessment. The O/C need not be discontinued for mildly abnormal smears and associated treatment. (Barrier contraception reduces the risk of abnormal smears and should be discussed.)

4. *Other problems*
   a) Breakthrough bleeding
      – check dose of oestrogen (increased) or progestogen (increased)

- change from phasic to continuous doses
- may be due to concurrent antibiotics (enzyme induction in liver)
b) Amenorrhoea
   - this is harmless: main problem is reassuring the woman she is not pregnant
   - if she *is* pregnant there is no evidence for O/C causing fetal abnormality
c) Cervical ectropion
d) Candida infection
e) Benign breast disease (less common on combined O/C)
f) Benign ovarian neoplasms (less common on combined O/C)
g) Benign hepatoma (more common on combined O/C (10–20 fold increase) but risk still only 1/100 000 users/year)

Effects of progestogens in *combined* pill:
- increased BP when oestrogen also given (i.e. *not* if POP given)
- increased arterial disease if oestrogens also given – mainly for norethisterone/levonorgestrel group, possibly due to:
   - metabolic effects – lipids – most increased
                        – HDL cholesterol – decreased
                        – blood sugar – increased

Prescribing   It is essential to be thoroughly familiar with at least three combined O/Cs – the choice is yours. *Examples* are:

1. With ethinyloestradiol 35 µg – Cilest (norgestimate)
                                – Bi- or Trinovum
                                  (norethisterone)
                                  (phasic pills)

2. With ethinyloestradiol 30 µg – Microgynon
                                  (levonorgestrel)
                                – Marvelon
                                  (desogestrel)
                                – Femodene
                                  (gestodene)

3. With ethinyloestradiol 20 µg – Mercilon
                                  (desogestrel)
                                – Loestrin 20
                                  (norethisterone)

Progestogens – The risks and benefits of third-generation progestogens (desogestrel, gestodene, norgestimate) *vs* second-generation progestogens (levonorgestrel, norethisterone) should be discussed with the woman:
- greater thromboembolic risk
- better effects on lipids
- less androgenic (better for acne, weight gain, mastalgia)
- use the 'ladder rung' model (JCC) and prescribe the lowest dose in each group
- use formulations which are themselves effective and do not require to be metabolised to an active form (e.g. levonorgestrel is preferred to norgestrel)

– *use high-dose oestrogens only when necessary* (concurrent drug therapy, e.g. for epilepsy/long-term antibiotics, etc.)

Contraindications to combined O/C

All situations should be judged individually.

Absolute contraindications:
– arterial/venous thrombosis
– ischaemic heart disease and cardiomyopathy
– close family relative (<45 years) with arterial or venous disease (may be familial lipid disorder)
– focal or crescendo migraine
– transient ischaemic attacks
– previous cerebral haemorrhage (increased BP raises risk)
– blood dyscrasias, thrombophilias or connective tissue disease (SLE, Factor V Leiden deficiency) which predispose to thrombosis
– active or recent liver disease
– cholestatic jaundice (on O/C or pregnancy)
– gallstones
– porphyria (many precipitate an attack)
– otosclerosis
– recent trophoblastic disease (OK when β-HCG is normal again)
– Crohn's disease (may relapse with hormonal treatments)
– pregnancy
– undiagnosed genital tract bleeding
– breast carcinoma or other oestrogen-dependent tumour

Relative contraindications:
– age >35 years (if combined with other factors)
– smoking
– family history of thromboembolic disease in first degree relative under 45 years
– hypertension
– immobilisation (long-term, e.g. wheelchair bound)
– hyperprolactinaemia
– diabetes (effect on glucose/arterial disease)
– splenectomy
– sickle cell disease
– chronic renal disease
– obesity (BMI >30 kg/m^2)

Notes:
1. The combined O/C should be stopped 1 month before *major* surgery (but can be continued before more minor procedures, e.g. sterilisation/D&C).
2. Varicose veins are *not* a contraindication in the absence of any thrombotic history or other predisposing factor.

Indications for stopping the combined pill

– emergence of a contraindication
– change in age or smoking habit
– diastolic pressure >95 mmHg (sustained)
– jaundice

- elective major surgery (1 month before)
- varicose vein surgery (1 month before)
- long-term immobilisation
- focal migraine
- swollen calf (venogram)
- suspected pulmonary embolism
- transient weakness (?CVA)
- disturbed speech (?CVA)
- visual disturbances (?TIA)
- a collapse (?TIA)

Notes

1. *Hypertension* develops in 5% of pill users after 5 years. The risk is increased if there is a history of hypertension in pregnancy, renal disease or a strong family history.

   If the BP rises above 160 mmHg systolic or 95 mmHg diastolic, the pill should be stopped. If the BP fails to return to normal within 6 months it needs investigating. No woman with unexplained hypertension should take the pill, and BP should be monitored every 6 months in *all* women on the pill.

2. *Fertility* is not impaired by the pill, although women who stop the pill can suffer a delay of a few months before the restoration of normal fertility. Post-pill amenorrhoea needs full investigation but nearly always responds to clomiphene.

3. The incidence of *gallstones* is slightly increased after 3 years on the pill.

4. *The metabolic effects* of the pill are:
   - increased cholesterol
   - increased triglycerides
   - increased renin substrate (hypertension)
   - increased platelet stickiness
   - enzyme induction

5. *Drug interactions.* Rifampicin, phenobarbitone, phenytoin and carbamazepine are enzyme-inducers and lower the plasma levels of ethinyloestradiol (EE). Women on these drugs should be prescribed a 50 µg pill.

   Ampicillin can lower the oestrogen levels (probably by decreasing gut flora that deconjugate ethinyloestradiol prior to reabsorption). Irregular bleeding may occur and pregnancies have been reported.

   Higher doses of insulin or warfarin may be needed.

6. *Depression* due to the pill sometimes responds to supplements of pyridoxine, 100 mg daily.

7. *The combined pill can also be used for*
   - dysmenorrhoea
   - ovulation pain
   - menorrhagia
   - endometriosis
   - functional ovarian cysts
   - regulation of periods (after disease excluded)

8. There is a decreased incidence of benign breast disease, ectopic pregnancies and carcinoma of the ovary and endometrium in women on the combined pill.

Note: The 1985 House of Lords ruling means it is legal to prescribe the pill to girls under 16 *without* their parents' consent.

◆ Progesterone-only pill (POP)

The following are in current UK usage:
- Microval/Norgeston – levonorgestrel 30 µg
- Neogest – norgestrel 75 µg (= levonorgestrel 37.5 µg)
- Micronor/Noriday – norethisterone 350 µg
- Femulen – ethynodiol diacetate 500 µg

The POP or mini-pill has a failure rate of 2% per year but this falls with age. Its main action is on cervical mucus (an 'oral barrier method') but it also makes the endometrium unreceptive and in some women inhibits ovulation.

It is contraindicated with a history of previous ectopic pregnancy or in those with an increased risk of ectopics, e.g. with a history of pelvic inflammatory disease or following tubal surgery (? slows tubal motility and increases the recurrence risk). Pregnancies occurring on the POP are more likely to be ectopic. There is no evidence of a tendency to thrombosis. The POP has no major undesirable side-effects, but is *contraindicated* in:
- previous ectopic pregnancy
- undiagnosed vaginal bleeding
- severe arterial disease (past or present)
- hypertriglyceridaemia
- hydatidiform mole (Both the combined O/C and POP should be avoided until HCG normal: research suggests earlier use doubles the likelihood of needing chemotherapy to prevent invasive choriocarcinoma.)
- carcinoma of the breast (theoretical risk)

Enzyme inducers (rifampicin, anticonvulsants) will reduce the contraceptive efficacy.

Uses
1. Contraception during lactation. The POP does not suppress lactation (although the 30 µg oestrogen pills probably do not suppress lactation either). It is excreted in minute amounts in breast milk but has no known adverse effects on the baby. Change to the combined pill, on the first day of a period, once breast feeding has stopped.
2. Contraception for women with troublesome oestrogenic side-effects from the combined pill, e.g.
   - fluid retention, weight gain
   - headache
   - chloasma
3. The POP can be used if the combined pill is contraindicated by:
   - migraine
   - thrombosis, embolus
   - liver disease
   - hypertension
   - diabetes
   - age over 35 and a smoker

High-density lipoprotein levels are not significantly altered by the POP. When the POP is prescribed for patients who have become hypertensive on the combined pill, the BP usually drops to normal.

In diabetics the POP may reduce the risks of arterial disease and of accelerating retinopathy.

4. For older women, the POP can be a very suitable method of contraception. A problem is knowing when the menopause is reached. Elevated FSH is probably diagnostic. Hot flushes or amenorrhoea may occur – the POP should be stopped and alternative methods used for at least a year.

Instructions

1. Take one tablet every day. A packet lasts 5–6 weeks. Start on day 1 of a period and use a sheath for 14 days while the effect builds up. The ideal time of day to take it depends on the woman's preferred time of intercourse: the peak action occurs after about 5 hours. Stress, however, that the POP must be taken at the same time each day – if more than 3 hours late on any day use a sheath for 14 days.

   If changing from the combined pill to the POP, start the day after the last pill.

2. Nausea, breast tenderness and breakthrough bleeding are common with the first packet but usually settle down.

3. If, after taking the pill, vomiting (within 2 hours) or diarrhoea (within 12 hours) occurs, take another pill.

Problems

1. It has a 2% failure rate per year in younger women.
2. It needs to be taken very accurately.
3. Erratic bleeding is thought to be more common on the POP.
   Three patterns exist:
   – normal cycles, ovulation occurs (40% of women)
   – shortened/erratic/frequent bleeds, due to rapid fluctuations of progesterone level or shortening of luteal phase (44% of women)
   – amenorrhoea or intermittent very light bleeds, ovaries quiescent and pregnancy risk very low (16% of women)
   Irregular bleeding is the most common reason for not liking the POP. It may be less on a higher dose (e.g. Femulen).
4. Missed periods. If there is a good chance of pregnancy stop the POP (the effect on the fetus is unknown). If pregnancy is excluded (examine and send urine test), it means that the woman has had an anovular cycle and that this low dose of hormone is inhibiting ovulation, making her extra safe. It probably means she will have an increased chance of later post-pill amenorrhoea (reversible with clomiphene).
5. Luteal cysts and abdominal pains occur occasionally.
6. Increased incidence of ectopics (0.1% of users).

◆ Injectables

There are two preparations:
– Depo-Provera 150 mg i.m. every 12 weeks (medroxyprogesterone)
– Noristerat 200 mg i.m. every 8 weeks (norethisterone oenanthate)

These preparations are available for long-term use in over 90 countries and are strongly supported by the WHO and the IPPF (International Planned Parenthood Federation) but only received FDA approval for the USA in 1992.

- less than 1% of women in the UK use a depot-injection preparation
- best given in the first few days of bleeding and then has immediate contraceptive effect
- postpartum: best given at 6 weeks; earlier administration causes more erratic and heavy bleeding
- after TOP: best given at day 7 (does not then interfere with bleeding due to RPOC)
- highly effective: failure rate is <1/100 women years
- no documented adverse effects on BP or gynaecological malignancy in humans
- could be more widely prescribed with benefit
- late attendance for follow-up injection – check not pregnant, or if only a few days late consider combined O/C or IUD insertion with repeat injection

Problems
- delayed return of fertility (but eventually normal)
- galactorrhoea may occur
- theoretical loss of bone density in amenorrhoeic women: long-term use (>5 years) depends on assessment of bone density, especially in amenorrhoeic patients

Contraindications are as for the POP, but injectables reliably inhibit ovulation so *protect* against ectopic pregnancy and functional ovarian cysts.

Other depot systems
1. *Norplant.* Released 1993 in the UK, but withdrawn recently, largely due to difficulties with removal. As effective as sterilisation. Some women will continue to have the implant in place until 2004. Six microtubules containing levonorgestrel in a slow release silastic 'carrier' base are implanted subdermally, usually into forearm, under local anaesthesia. Efficacy persists for 5 years. Remove as required.
   - failure rate 0.2/100 women years
   - delivers a steady daily dose (depot injections deliver an exponentially falling dose; oral POP delivers a highly fluctuating dose every 24 hours)
   - fertility returns promptly
   - side-effects similar to POP
   (New market releases of similar 1- and 3-year systems are being developed.)
2. *Mirena* intrauterine system. A levonorgestrel-releasing IUD: (20 µg/24 hrs). Highly effective contraceptive with a very low ectopic pregnancy rate (in contrast to previous 'Progestasert'). Lasts 5–7 years. In contrast to other intrauterine devices, Mirena reduces both menstrual blood loss (it is now also licensed for first-line treatment of menorrhagia) and pelvic inflammatory disease. It also inhibits ovulation in a majority of women. Erratic bleeding for the first 6 months can be expected, often followed by amenorrhoea. (Also said to be effective as the progestogen component of combined HRT, e.g. with transdermal oestrogen patches/gel or implants, but not yet licensed for this use in the UK.)

3. Vaginal rings – levonorgestrel in silastic ring. Other progestogens under study.

◆ Non-medicated intrauterine device (IUD)

Approximately 5% of women in the UK use an IUD for contraception. In 1988 there were an estimated 85 million users worldwide. In the Far East it is a very popular method, with approximately 60 million users in China alone.

The IUD works by interfering with fertilisation and implantation. Devices are now usually copper-bearing (limited years of use), but older designs were inert. The newest development has been the progestogen-bearing device. Copper devices generally cost under £10 each, but the Mirena IUS costs almost £100.

1. Inert devices: tend to be larger (more side-effects) but may remain in place for many years, therefore a popular choice for Third World countries (e.g. the Lippes loop.)
2. Progestogen-bearing – see the Mirena IUS above.
3. Copper-bearing devices (the following available in UK):
   - Multiload Cu250 and Cu250 Short (replace every 3 years)
   - Nova-T (replace every 5 years)
   - GyneFix 380 (change at 5 years)

   Failure rate declines with increased duration of use but is approximately 0.5–2%, often due to unrecognised expulsion of the device, especially in the first year of use.

   Secret of IUD success lies in:
   - correct insertion: timing and technique
   - accurate measurement of uterine size
   - correct choice of device (size)

   Best time to insert is day 4–14 of cycle. Removal can be during a period or at any time provided there is 7 days of alternative contraception cover.

Advantages of the IUD
- useful for the forgetful or if the pill is contraindicated
- long-term protection, more effective than barrier methods
- local action with no metabolic effects
- immediate action that is also immediately reversible
- no day-to-day motivation needed (although high motivation is needed to have it inserted) and positive action needed to reverse it
- no supplies needed
- does not spoil the spontaneity of sex
- can be used when breastfeeding
- can be used for postcoital contraception (within 5 days)
- low mortality rate (and no evidence of increased endometrial carcinoma)
- relatively inexpensive

Disadvantages/risks
- expulsion and unwanted pregnancy
- perforation (at insertion)
- malposition increases symptoms and failure rate
- pelvic infection (not with Mirena IUS)
- pain and heavier periods (not with Mirena IUS)

- IUD does not *cause* ectopic pregnancy, but it is not protective either: it may appear that more pregnancies are ectopic but overall, the risk of pregnancy is reduced (both intra- and extrauterine). Ectopic risk is linked more to pelvic infection than to IUD usage
- lost threads – exclude pregnancy, sound cervical canal, ultrasound
  - $\pm$ X-ray to localise IUD elsewhere in abdomen
  - laparoscopy + removal

Particular problems:
- previous ectopic pregnancy: advise another method – no specifically increased risk but any pregnancy may be tubal, risking fertility
- STD: screen prior to insertion. Avoid insertion until treated
- uterine anomaly/fibroids malposition
- Wilson's disease: precludes use of Cu-bearing devices
- known cardiac/valve disease or other prosthesis
- diabetes (relative contraindication)
- contraindicated in HIV or immunosuppressed patients

Cautionary note: Insertion may cause vagal shock – always have airway, O_2 and atropine (0.6 mg i.m.) available. Also:
- mefenamic acid (pre- or post-insertion use)
- diazepam can be useful
- adrenaline 1 : 1000 (1 ml s.c.) for allergic collapse

Method of insertion

1. Bimanual for position of uterus (anteverted or retroverted) to exclude pregnancy and screen for ovarian masses.
2. Smear if needed (screening).
3. Swab cervix with antiseptic.
4. Apply tenaculum forceps to steady the cervix.
5. Pass a sound.
6. Insert IUD of correct size using no-touch technique.
7. Repass the sound to check IUD is not lying in the cervical canal (if it is, remove and replace).
8. The woman should rest for 10–20 minutes.

The following points must be explained to the patient:
1. Continue to use alternative contraception for the first 6 weeks (when expulsion rate is highest). The woman is seen again at 6 weeks to check the position. In the meantime she should check the threads every week. Most women find this straightforward, but always check by speculum examination that the threads (but not the device!) are seen coming through at the os.
2. Tampons can be used provided the threads are checked when one is removed. Intercourse can be resumed immediately.
3. Most women get crampy pains for 2 or 3 days after insertion and should be warned of this. This is more likely if insertion was painful (treat with Bucospan).
4. Some irregular spotting often occurs throughout the first cycle. The periods, particularly the first two or three, will be heavier. The normal discharge also tends to be a bit heavier.
5. Annual follow-up is necessary for a smear (which will also pick up any actinomycosis) and to exclude anaemia if the IUD causes heavy periods.

Use close to menopause: IUD is an ideal method if menstrual loss is not erratic, in which case investigate in the usual way for pathology. Leave IUD for 12 months after last period, then remove.

◆ Barrier methods

All these are advantageous for reducing the incidence of STDs.
– diaphragm or cap
– female condom
– male condom

Diaphragm About 3% of married women in the UK use the diaphragm, but it is more popular in the US where women are more concerned about complications of the pill and the IUD.

Major role is to keep spermicide in ideal location plus some slowing of sperm transfer to cervix.

It has many *advantages*:
– effective: the failure rate is 2–3% per year but falls with age and with greater experience of the method
– no systemic side-effects
– lowest mortality (including from terminations for failures) apart from vasectomy
– protection against carcinoma of the cervix
– spontaneity not spoiled (unlike the sheath) because it is inserted beforehand and neither partner feels it during intercourse
– spermicide may help vaginal dryness

The *problems* with the method: good motivation is necessary (it must be used *every* time); some women find the idea of inserting a diaphragm messy or unpleasant, a certain amount of dexterity is necessary (arthritis or weakness may make it impossible) and allergy to the spermicide can develop occasionally. Although diaphragms can be bought over the counter, they need to be fitted initially by a doctor or nurse. A diaphragm that is too large may cause mechanical urethritis and, left in too long, possibly predisposes to infection.

The diaphragm is a neat hemisphere of rubber with a flat metal spring in the rim. It works by holding spermicide near the cervix. A wide range of sizes are available but, in practice, the correct size will be a diameter of 65–85 mm (increasing in 5 mm steps except for 72.5 mm). The principle is to fit the largest diaphragm that is comfortable.

Fitting
1. VE to examine the adnexae and cervix (screening) and to exclude cystocele, prolapse or poor vaginal tone, which will prevent retention of the diaphragm. Retroversion of the uterus makes no difference (although fitting the diaphragm into the posterior fornix can be more difficult).
2. Assess the size required by inserting the index finger into the posterior fornix and measuring the distance to the pubis.
3. A set of measuring rings can be used but a set of diaphragms is better. Choose a diaphragm of about the right size (the dome can be up or down – usually up) and compress the ring between finger and thumb.

Insert along the posterior vaginal wall until it is in the posterior fornix. The anterior rim is then pushed up behind the pubis.

4. The diaphragm fits diagonally across the vagina and covers the cervix and most of the anterior vaginal wall. If it does not cover the cervix, choose a larger size. If it causes discomfort, choose a smaller size (it should not distend the vaginal walls).

5. Next the woman is taught how to insert the diaphragm, either squatting or with a foot on a chair: 'Compress the rim then push it downwards rather than upwards as far as possible, then push the anterior rim up behind the bone with your forefinger. Next check that the neck of the womb is covered by feeling it (like the tip of the nose) through the diaphragm.'

6. Demonstrate how to put cream on the diaphragm. A 10 cm strip is needed to inactivate an ejaculate and most of it should be put on the surface in contact with the os.

   Provide the woman with a practice diaphragm of the correct size and see her in a week, with it in place (to have the position checked). During that week she should:
   - practise inserting it with a spermicide
   - practise wearing it during the day and during sex, but
   - not rely on it for contraception

7. The following week, the position is checked and if the size is correct (no discomfort, not dislodged during sex or expelled by straining), a diaphragm of that size is prescribed.

   Pain (backache, urethritis) is a sign that the diaphragm is too large and often the rim will be bent. Occasionally the diaphragm is too small and jams between the cervix and pubis.

8. The diaphragm comes in a plastic box (like a powder compact). Spermicidal cream must be put on the diaphragm before insertion. A pessary is necessary if intercourse is delayed for 2 hours or repeated (they take 5 minutes to melt).

   The diaphragm can be bought over the counter but is free on prescription, e.g. Type A Diaphragm with flat metal spring (available sizes 55–95 mm) + Duragel spermicidal cream 100 g × 3 or Orthoforms pessaries (15) × 3.

The following points need to be explained (both verbally and with a leaflet if possible):

1. It must be used on *every* occasion and *always with a spermicide*.

2. It can be inserted at any convenient time before intercourse (the ideal would be routine insertion every night). If intercourse takes place over 2 hours after insertion insert additional spermicide (pessary or foam). If intercourse is repeated, insert additional spermicide.

3. Leave in place for at least 6 hours after intercourse. On removal rinse in soap and water and dry. Do not leave in longer than 24 hours.

4. Walking about or urinating will not displace the diaphragm. A bowel movement may displace it, so check afterwards that it is still covering the cervix.

5. If a period starts with it in place, it does not matter (the blood will trickle around the edges): leave it in for the full 6 hours and use a tampon as normal.
6. Inspect occasionally for holes and keep the rim circular. Do not stretch it and never boil it and it should last 2 years.
7. Have the size re-checked:
   - if weight changes by 10 lb (5 kg)
   - 6 weeks postpartum (even a section)
   - if vaginal surgery is performed
   - every 12 months

Cervical/vault caps Stay in place by suction. Poor failure rate is due to poor compliance with strict use of method, compounded by poor teaching by medical/nursing staff of correct technique.

Female condom (e.g. Femidom) First marketed in 1992. Approximately 17 cm long with 70 mm external ring and softer 60 mm ring at upper closed end. Useful if high STD risk. Thicker than male condoms so less liable to 'split'. Awaiting greater acceptability/popularity and remains expensive compared with the male condom. Failure rate so far unclear, but probably quite effective if users are well motivated.

Male condom In 1544 Fallopius advocated the use of a linen sheath to protect against venereal disease.

The condom is widely used and has several *advantages*:
- highly reliable (if used properly), especially those including a spermicide
- no health risks
- easily available, no need to see a health professional
- protective against STD
- possibly decreased carcinoma of the cervix

Used by well-informed and well-motivated couples, failure rates as low as 0.4 per 100 women years have been reported; used incorrectly, the failure rate is 20–30. The condom has the disadvantage that it is coitus-related and therefore of low acceptability for some couples. Allergy (to latex) can develop.

Instructions for use:
1. Use on every occasion.
2. Use before any genital contact.
3. Always use with a spermicide.
4. The man must hold it on when withdrawing.
5. Use once only, before the expiry date.

The condom can be prescribed on FP10, can be obtained free from Family Planning Clinics, and is widely available in shops or from vending machines in clubs etc.

◆ Spermicides

Must be used with all barrier methods. Consist of an inert base (usually water soluble) and an active component – nonoxinol '9' is the most common. (Active component often already present in male condoms.)

◆ Contraceptive sponge

Impregnated with nonoxinol '9' and mainly effective as a carrier of the spermicide to the cervix. Failure rates as high as 25% have been reported.

◆ Natural methods

Natural methods of family planning rely on abstinence during the fertile part of the cycle. This can be calculated using a calendar or recognised by symptoms or temperature methods (or both).

These methods, especially in combination, can provide very effective contraception if used by well-motivated couples. Some couples practise withdrawal during the fertile phase of the cycle, however, making the method much less reliable.

The calendar method
This method is based on the fact that ovulation always occurs 14 days before a period. In a regular 28-day cycle the unsafe period has been found to be days 10–18. This is because:

- ovulation can vary around day 14
- the ovum survives 1 day
- sperm in the female reproductive tract survives 3 days

Ideally, the unsafe period should be stretched to allow for the longest and shortest cycles in the last 12 months. *If a cycle is short*, e.g. only 25 days, the follicular phase must be 3 days shorter than usual, so intercourse becomes unsafe 3 days earlier than usual (i.e. days 7–18 instead of 10–18); *If a cycle is long*, e.g. 32 days, the follicular phase is 4 days longer than usual, so intercourse remains unsafe for 4 extra days (i.e. days 10–22 instead of 10–18).

Note: The method is useless if periods are irregular, or the cycle length varies by more than 10 days.

Ovulatory signs/ temperature chart methods
Ovulation can be detected by:
- temperature rise
- ovulatory cascade of mucus. The cervical secretions become watery and can be pulled out into a thread (spin-barkheit), the 'Billing's method'

Note: Intercourse should not occur until 3 days after ovulation has been detected by these methods.

◆ Postcoital contraception

This method acts between intercourse and implantation (methods acting after implanation but before menstruation have a different ethical perspective for some women).

PCC is legal and approved by the DoH. Historically PCC has always been practised, with formal drug usage beginning in the 1960s using stilboestrol (DES). Because of the fetal effects of DES, ethinyloestradiol preparations are preferred.

Insertion (within a maximum of 5 days) of an IUD is also successful.

Regimens

1. Hormonal or 'Yuzpe' method: begin course within 72 hours (at most) of unprotected intercourse; earlier treatment is more effective. Two tablets, each containing 250 μg levonorgestrel and 50 μg ethinyloestradiol, followed 12 hours later by two more (e.g. Ovran). Unsuitable if there is a history of thrombosis or focal migraine at time of request. If vomiting occurs within 2 hours, repeat with a further two tablets together with an anti-emetic, or consider IUD insertion.
2. If oestrogens are contraindicated, use levonorgestrel 750 μg stat + 750 μg 12 hours later.
3. Higher doses of oestrogen can be used alone, but cause more side-effects with prolonged nausea/vomiting.

After postcoital contraception, patients must be advised that:
– the next period may be early or late (check pregnancy test)
– they must use barrier contraception until next period
– pain/bleeding must be reported promptly

If PCC fails: No evidence for teratogenesis (yet) but most women will request TOP (and be accepted).

◆ Sterilisation

Sterilisation of one partner is a simple and reliable method of contraception that is becoming increasingly popular. It is ideal for the stable couple who are absolutely certain that whatever happens, they will not want any more children and who have several years of potential fertility ahead of them (it may not be worthwhile if the woman is nearing the menopause).

Although it is expensive, it is cost-effective in community terms. A woman with an IUD for 10 years has a theoretical 1 in 10 chance of an unwanted pregnancy followed by either termination (expensive) or childbirth which, with increasing age, is associated with increased perinatal and maternal mortality.

Sterilisation is essentially a destructive operation and counselling is important to avoid years of bitter regret. The GP is in the ideal position to be sure the couple are making a mature, informed decision and to advise a hospital colleague.

The couple should be seen together so they both clearly understand the procedure and its implications.

The following points need to be discussed:
– Alternative methods
– Irreversibility
– Male or female?
– Female sterilisation
– Vasectomy
– Side-effects

- Failure rate
- Consent

1. *Alternative methods* will usually have been considered by the couple, but the GP should mention them (particularly POP, diaphragm, IUD) and compare their merits or dismerits with sterilisation. The advantages of sterilisation should be discussed as well as the disadvantages.

2. *Irreversibility*. The procedure must be considered irreversible. Reversal is still only successful in 50%. In the female it requires complicated microsurgery (time-consuming and expensive) and increases the risk of an ectopic ten-fold. In the male, reversibility is technically easy but only 50% achieve fertility, possibly because anti-sperm antibodies have developed. Therefore the GP must enquire about factors which might make the request for reversal likely:
   - both young (or one partner much older)
   - recent or sudden decision
   - psychiatric history
   - stability of marriage (sexual, social, financial)
   - number and ages of children (?under 1 year)
   - medical condition of children

3. *Male or female?* The couple will usually have already decided but may ask the doctor for advice.

   Preferably it should be performed on the woman if she has health reasons for avoiding future pregnancies (although there can be major surgical risks due to pelvic adhesions or anaesthetic risks). History or examination may reveal indications for a hysterectomy:
   - fibroids
   - menorrhagia
   - abnormal smear
   - prolapse
   - ovarian mass

   If for one partner sterilisation symbolises genital trauma (despite reassurance) it is best avoided.

   Vasectomy is quicker but takes 3 months to have contraceptive effect confirmed. The risks of failure or complications (haemorrhage, infection) are equal. Vasectomy is easier to reverse and has a lower mortality of 1 in 100 000, compared with 10 in 10 000 for female sterilisation.

4. *Female sterilisation*. This can be achieved by:
   - laparoscopy (clips usually in UK, also rings or diathermy)
   - laparotomy (Pomeroy or Irving techniques)
   - hysterectomy
   - vaginal approaches (culdoscopy, colpotomy)

   Laparoscopic sterilisation using clips is usually the method of choice. The fibreoptic laparoscope is introduced through a 1cm incision in the lower umbilical fold and the clip applicator is inserted through a separate incision. It is a difficult operation technically, but only a small area of tube is damaged, causing less postoperative pain and good potential for reversibility. The failure rate is about 1 in 500. The Filshie clip is made of titanium and lined with silicone rubber which expands as the fallopian tube necroses. It is simple to apply. (The Hulka-Clemens clip is an alternative, used less commonly now.)

Stopping the pill prior to this type of surgery is *not* necessary and the woman should continue the packet until the end of the cycle before relying on sterilisation. It is usually performed under GA: she is allowed home when she is recovered, with analgesia (usually the same day) and is off work for about a week.

Rings cause more postoperative pain from the strangulated loop of tube (1 in 500 fail). Diathermy is irreversible (4 cm of tube destroyed) and gut can be damaged (1 in 500 fail).

Laparotomy and tubal ligation via a suprapubic incision is necessary if the woman is very obese or has pelvic adhesions. This can also be performed after elective caesarean section or within 72 hours of delivery (via an incision at the level of the fundus) if the woman made the decision early in pregnancy. Post-abortal sterilisation should be avoided for emotional reasons (and higher failure rate).

The original Pomeroy ligation has a 1 in 500 failure rate (up to 1 in 50 on vascular postpartum tubes). The Irving technique (in which the proximal stump is buried in the myometrium) has a failure rate of 1 in 1000.

Excised tube should be sent for histology (to prove it is fallopian tube).

Culdoscopy or *colpotomy* is rarely performed and the insertion of tubal plugs via a transcervical hysteroscope remains experimental.

5. *Vasectomy* is a simple and safe outpatient procedure performed under local anaesthetic, and takes about 20 minutes. Bilateral short incisions are made high in the scrotum, each vas is dissected free, 2 cm excised and the ends doubled back to prevent recanalisation.

A GA may be necessary if there is a varicocele or hydrocele. (Ligation of the vas can also be performed during a herniorrhaphy or prostatectomy.)

Postoperatively an athletic support should be worn day and night for a week, to avoid pain. Scrotal bruising often looks dramatic but usually subsides in a few weeks without treatment. The risk of haematoma is decreased by taking 2 days off work with no heavy lifting. Occasional complications are:
- haematoma (3%: ice packs, drain if large)
- infection (antibiotics)
- epididymo-orchitis (rarely)

The volume of ejaculate is unchanged. Sperm clearance takes about 20 ejaculations. Two negative counts at 12 and 14 weeks should be obtained before abandoning other methods of contraception. Persistent sperm occurs rarely, due to operative error or double vas, and this requires re-exploration. The failure rate (1–3 per 1000) is due to recanalisation.

Vasectomy is cheaper than female sterilisation and requires less expertise, equipment and time both to perform and reverse.

6. The *mortality* of female sterilisation, which involves opening the peritoneum, is about 1 in 10000 and is much lower for male sterilisation (1 in 100000). *Complications* of infection or haemorrhage arise occasionally, with equal frequency in males and females.

Many people fear effects on their masculinity or femininity, libido, sexual performance, volume of ejaculate, etc., and explanation with diagrams of the mechanical nature of the procedure is important. A common question asked is about what happens to the eggs/sperm (which are absorbed by normal body processes).

Some women complain of heavier periods and should be warned of this if they will be stopping the pill. In most others it is probably coincidental dysfunctional bleeding and there is no evidence that sterilisation has any endocrine effects. Long-term follow-up of vasectomy patients has revealed an increase in anti-sperm antibodies but no harmful systemic effects.

7. *Failure rate*. The couple must be aware that sterilisation can fail (1–3 per 1000), due to recanalisation or poor operative technique. After tubal occlusion about 20% of such pregnancies are ectopic.

8. Written informed *consent* must be obtained from the person being sterilised, who must be over 16. The consent of the partner is not legally necessary but should be obtained where possible. If the decision is uncertain, sterilisation should normally be postponed because it can worsen a poor relationship or lead to regret and requests for reversal (most purchasing authorities no longer fund reversal procedures, some no longer fund sterilisation either). Photographic evidence of correct clip placement (from video laparoscopy) can reduce litigation attempts after failed sterilisation.

◆ Psychosexual counselling

The incidence of sexual problems is unknown. Surveys reveal that 15% of men and 30% of women feel they have sexual problems of some kind. Referral rate for counselling, however, is only about 6 cases per 10 000 population (i.e. 1–2 cases per GP) per year. There are three landmarks in the development of our present attitudes to sex:

1. In 1949 Kinsey published statistical reports showing that sexual activity (both homo- and heterosexual) was much more widespread than had generally been assumed. He saw sex as a powerful innate force that demanded expression.

   Sex is of course extremely important to most people, and many people view the loss of sexual function as more important than losing an eye or a limb.

2. In 1986 Masters and Johnson published *Human Sexual Response*. Using volunteers in a laboratory setting, they analysed the physical events of sexual intercourse and demonstrated that women also have orgasms and that they are always due to clitoral stimulation. They developed a method of therapy to treat sexual problems, but concentrated on the physical rather than the emotional aspects of sex.

   Ignorance about the plain facts of the anatomy and physiology of sexual intercourse still causes many psychosexual problems.

3. In 1974 Alex Comfort published the *Joy of Sex* and emphasised that sex should be recreational and not just a battle to achieve as many orgasms as possible. He pointed out that sex has a therapeutic and relaxing effect that drains away aggression.

Inherent in this view of sex as an enjoyable act is the assumption that both partners have communicated about the rules. Social myths about what each partner *should* feel and do, together with lack of communication about what each partner would *like* to do, are the commonest causes of psychosexual problems. Non-judgemental information in written or CD-ROM format can be useful in educating couples and individuals about aspects of human sexuality without the need to discuss the problems face to face with health professionals.

Counselling is a form of psychotherapy. Lasting change can be achieved by listening and talking. To be effective, two things are required of the therapist:
a) The right sort of personality. A therapist can rarely help someone he does not like. He has to feel empathy and respect (even respect for bizarre fantasies) and must form a relationship with the person or couple. Otherwise behaviour is unlikely to change.
b) A therapist must be willing to interact and discuss/express his or her own feelings.

Given that the therapist is sensitive and has healthy attitudes to sex, exploring the patient's true feelings about the subject is the best way to lead them to a useful new understanding and awareness. This demands personal honesty from the therapist, who must also have no preconceived ideas about the likely areas of conflict causing the problem. The Masters and Johnson method involves giving the couple tasks to do at home, then counselling on emotional reactions and communication.

In practice many psychosexual problems can be resolved by simple discussion and common sense.

No two people are the same. To help a couple with a sexual problem, a doctor must understand his own attitudes, be willing to listen sympathetically and be able to offer a working vocabulary, e.g. 'do you have problems with lack of sexual appetite, poor lubrication, having a climax, ejaculating too soon, keeping an erection?', etc. Depending on the problem, a very detailed history (and sometimes examination) is usually necessary – physical illness must not be missed. The following is merely a check list:

Psychosexual history

1. *The problem*. It usually falls into one of the following categories:
   – libido
   – stimulation
   – intercourse
   – orgasm
2. *Intercourse*. Has it ever been enjoyable? Frequency, pain or difficulty (impotence, premature ejaculation, vaginismus). Frequency of orgasm. Contraception.
3. *Periods*. (Does she use tampons or towels?) Any infertility. Obstetric history is very important (e.g. termination, stillbirths, puerperal difficulties, attitudes to breastfeeding).
4. *Sexual history*. Attitudes, derived from family and education. Fantasies or recurring dreams. Masturbation. Previous sexual experiences (heterosexual, homosexual, incest, rape).

5. *Personal history*. Friends, relationships, school, career, achievement, religious and moral attitudes. Marital or extramarital relationships.
6. *Social history*. (Family, housing, job.)
7. *Past medical, drug or psychiatric history*.

The GP is often the ideal person to help a couple with sexual problems. Patients often disguise the problem, sometimes for years, and the possibility of psychosexual problems should be considered in patients with multiple symptoms.

Many psychosexual problems are solved using simple common sense to improve communications. However, not every couple can be helped: some simply no longer have any love for each other, some have complex difficulties that defy easy resolution, some have deep-seated personality problems.

Counselling is time-consuming. Patients can be referred to trained psychosexual counsellors via a Family Planning Clinic or Relate.

Psychosexual problems

The problems are categorised here into:
1. Physical causes
2. The relationship
3. Ignorance
4. Social myths
5. Fear of failure
6. Failure

1. Physical causes

These are usually obvious, but nevertheless must not be overlooked. Superficial dyspareunia may be due to candidiasis, trichomoniaisis or atrophic changes. Sometimes an episiotomy scar or congenital abnormality requires plastic surgery.

Deep dyspareunia may be due to endometriosis or chronic salpingitis and may be an indication for laparoscopy. Sometimes chronic cervicitis causes deep pain and requires cryocautery.

Premature ejaculation can rarely be due to urinary infection, prostatitis or neurological disease.

Impotence is usually psychological but consider:
– depression
– alcohol
– drugs (hypotensives, thiazides, anxiolytics, steroids, cimetidine)
– diabetic neuropathy (50% over age 60)
– pituitary tumour (either causing *hyperprolactinaemia or hypopituitarism with low FSH and LH: serum testosterone* will be low in both cases)

An intracavernosal injection of an α-blocking drug, e.g. phenoxybenzamine can be self-administered and causes an erection lasting for several hours.

Loss of libido can be due to general ill-health, e.g. hypothyroidism, chronic renal failure (improves with dialysis) or psychiatric illness, e.g. schizophrenia.

2. The relationship

Sexual problems often dissolve once the relationship between the couple improves. Conversely, sexual problems cannot be solved while a relationship remains poor.

The problem is nearly always one of *poor communication*. Conflicts about children, relatives, job, etc. may be unresolved. One partner may be suffering low self-esteem, either mental (depression), physical (obesity, postnatal, postmenopausal, coronary, colostomy, mastectomy, hysterectomy) or social (unemployment, isolation).

The doctor can offer guidelines for re-establishing communication, e.g. setting time aside for discussion and openly stating emotional feelings. The doctor often somehow acts as a catalyst, and simply discussing the problems with the couple may be all that is needed.

3. Ignorance

Ignorance about the basic anatomy and physiology involved is still common. Before explaining anything find out what is not known.

Foreplay and mutual stimulation are often hampered by attitudes such as 'men automatically know what to do', 'women should be passive' or 'it's wrong to talk during sex'. The doctor can encourage sexual communication by suggesting that they lead their partner's hand to touch sensitive areas and tell each other what they feel like.

There may be ignorance about the need for both clitoral and vaginal stimulation and for female lubrication. There may be strange fantasies about what the vagina is like inside (e.g. 'like tissue paper'), which may be dispelled by vaginal examination and explanation (ideally with the partner present) and by teaching the woman to examine herself.

Only the doctor can examine someone physically and he should never waste the opportunity of saying 'everything is normal'.

4. Social myths

Social myths still abound and most of them are variants of the following:
- 'Nice women don't do it'
- 'Real men don't show their feelings'

Inappropriate feelings, originating from parental, school or religious attitudes have often been retained. The doctor, as a similar figure of authority, is in a good position to reverse these and to *'give permission'* for more healthy feelings, for masturbation, oral sex or whatever the couple enjoy doing together. Merely discussing sexual matters openly is a form of permission giving.

5. Fear of failure

This always develops when there is sexual tension. Once the above problems have been resolved, anxiety about performance can be reduced by redefining 'success' simply as shared pleasure. If both partners are enjoying the experience, it does not matter how aroused each partner becomes relative to the other.

A simple way to reduce performance pressure is to ban intercourse for a while and have regular sessions of mutual caressing when demands for intercourse are not made – the *'sensate focus' technique* of Masters and Johnson. The couple should be encouraged to say what they are enjoying, so the partner knows that what they are doing is enjoyable for the other.

6. Failure

Temporary failure of intercourse may be due to tiredness, prying children or a creaking bed! More persistent problems are:
- premature ejaculation
- impotence

- vaginismus
- poor lubrication
- anorgasmia

Premature ejaculation is due to loss of voluntary control over ejaculation. Usually the man is trying to take his mind off his feelings in the mistaken belief that this will help prolong intercourse. He has to be taught to concentrate on recognising the pre-ejaculatory sensation. The best method of overcoming the problem is the *'squeeze technique'*. He signals to the woman just before ejaculation and she pinches the glans for about 30 seconds until the sensation goes away. As he gets better control he will learn to stop every so often during intercourse.

Impotence is usually psychological (guilt, low self-esteem, marital conflict) and this is confirmed if the man can have erections at other times, e.g. early morning, by masturbation or with other women. Simple counselling often relieves the problem.

Vaginismus is often due to unreasonable guilt feelings or fears of pain or damage, based on ignorance or fantasies, and can often be relieved by patient explanation, examination and by teaching self-examination. Graded dilators for use at home may be helpful. Sometimes it is due to deep-seated rejection of adult status: this requires prolonged psychotherapy.

Poor lubrication is usually due to inadequate stimulation by the man, but KY jelly is sometimes useful. Exclude atrophic vaginitis.

Anorgasmia: some women enjoy sex without ever achieving orgasm. The man may feel inadequate because he cannot 'give' the woman an orgasm. Often it is because she is not sufficiently relaxed to 'let herself go' completely.

Male impotence and Viagra

A systemic treatment for erectile dysfunction, sildenafil (Viagra), 25–50 mg orally (up to 100 mg depending on response) is available on NHS prescription for specific indications:
- neurological problems — diabetes, multiple sclerosis, Parkinson's disease, polio, spina bifida or severe spinal cord injury, rare single gene disorders
- men receiving dialysis for renal failure
- after renal transplant surgery
- after radical pelvic surgery, prostatic cancer surgery and severe pelvic injury
- men who were receiving NHS treatment for erectile dysfunction with alprostadil (MUSE, Caverject, Viridal) when the guidelines for NHS use of Viagra were announced on 14 September 1998.

Systemic side-effects include headache, flushing, tachycardia and chest pain. Sildenafil is strictly contraindicated in men taking nitrates. It must be used with caution in men with penile deformity (Peyronie's disease), hypercoagulable states, and liver disease.

There is considerable non-NHS usage of Viagra, and patients can purchase limited supplies for personal use. Deaths have been reported, mainly due to CVS effects and with excess dosage. Trials on its use in women are underway.

4. Obstetrics

Maternity care is a true multidisciplinary specialty, involving GP, midwife, obstetrician, paediatrician, anaesthetist, and the mother herself. Expectations are high with all concerned wanting a perfect baby and a happy, healthy mother.

The following definitions are important.

◆ Maternal mortality

Maternal death is defined as: the death of a woman while pregnant or within 42 days of termination of pregnancy (i.e. delivery, TOP or miscarriage) from any cause related to or aggravated by the pregnancy and its management, but not from accidental or incidental causes. The rate is expressed as *deaths/100 000 maternities*. This is different from the terminology used when calculating death rates in *early* pregnancy, when the total number of *estimated pregnancies* is the denominator.

- *maternities* are mothers delivered of a liveborn infant (at any gestation) or a stillborn infant after 24 weeks. (UK maternities in 1994–96 were reported at 2 197 640.)
- *estimated pregnancies* are the number of maternities plus legal terminations, hospital-treated spontaneous abortions <24 weeks, and ectopics. (The figure is adjusted for confounding factors and for the UK stood at 2 914 600 in 1994–96.)

Deaths are divided into:
- direct (an obstetric complication)
- indirect (exacerbation of a previous condition, or a new condition arising and aggravated by, but not due to, the pregnancy)
- late (direct and indirect deaths between 42 days and 1 year after pregnancy)
- fortuitous (unconnected with the pregnancy process, e.g. RTA)

Since 1952 a 3-yearly report called the *Confidential Enquiry into Maternal Deaths in England and Wales* has analysed all maternal deaths and considered the findings of obstetricians, anaesthetists and pathologists who review each case anonymously. The report focuses particularly on detection of 'substandard care' and is one of the earliest (and best) examples of clinical audit.

The maternal mortality rate has reduced dramatically since reporting began: in 1952 maternal deaths accounted for 40% of all female deaths in the 15–44 year age group. Maternal death now accounts for 7/1000 female deaths in this age group, a figure which has remained constant since the 1982–84 report.

The original dramatic fall was largely due to improvements in general maternal health, but also to improvements in maternity services generally:
- improved social conditions and health
- social services provisions
- antibiotics
- blood transfusion
- safer surgery
- improved anaesthesia
- more hospital deliveries
- falling parity

The most recent triennial report was published in November 1998 and covers 1994–96. It differs from previous reports in considering not only deaths formally reported to the enquiry, but also another 67 cases (identified from death certificates for example). The report identified 376 maternal deaths (12.2/100 000 maternities) – without the additional cases ascertained via the Office of National Statistics, the figure would have been 309 (9.9/100 000) – unchanged from the previous report. There were 134 direct, 134 indirect, and 72 late deaths. There were 36 fortuitous deaths. (The last three triennial reports covered the whole of the UK, whereas previous reports were for England and Wales only; percentages for the whole UK compare closely with those in previous England and Wales reports.) Maternal mortality rate varies between regions (as does PNM).

Causes of death

The causes of the 134 *direct deaths* were:
1. Thromboembolism (48)
2. Hypertensive disorders (20)
3. Amniotic fluid embolism (17)
4. Early pregnancy deaths (15)
   - ectopic (12)
   - miscarriage (2)
   - TOP (1)
5. Sepsis (14)

These 5 causes account for >85% of all direct maternal deaths.
6. Haemorrhage (12)
7. Other (7)
   - including 5 due to genital tract trauma
8. Anaesthesia (1)

Thromboembolism remains the leading cause, now at a rate of 21.8/1 000 000 maternities, higher than in the previous three reports (**Note**: 38% of fatal thromboembolism cases occurred *before* 24 weeks gestation.) Hypertension accounts for deaths in 9.1/1 000 000 maternities, a similar figure to those in previous reports, whereas haemorrhage caused fewer deaths than in previous reports. Although amniotic fluid embolism is rare, it continues to cause a substantial number of deaths. Anaesthetic deaths have greatly reduced, with only one death directly attributable (0.5/1 000 000) maternities.

Of the *indirect causes* of maternal death, cardiac and psychiatric causes are highlighted for attention.

Once again, *substandard care* was identified in many deaths, mainly –
– Not recognising warning signs:
　failure of junior staff to refer to a senior
　failure of GPs to refer to hospital
– Failure of senior staff:
　not attending, inappropriate delegation
　not referring to, or seeking advice from, other specialists early enough when appropriate
– Lack of clear guidelines for major emergencies such as eclampsia, haemorrhage, pulmonary embolism
– Lack of teamwork

◆ Perinatal mortality (PNM)

The perinatal mortality rate is defined as: the number of stillbirths plus the number of neonatal deaths in the first week, expressed per 1000 *total* births (i.e. both live births and stillbirths).

PNM has fallen steadily:
– around 500/1000 in deprived areas in the 1850s
– 35/1000 in 1958
– 11/1000 in 1986
– 8.2/1000 in 1997
– 7.9/1000 in 1998

The 1997/98 figures (from CESDI) are for England, Wales and N. Ireland. The rate in the 1990s has not changed dramatically, although the inclusion of gestations between 24–28 weeks since 1992 might have been expected to affect the figures. Several other countries have much lower rates (e.g. Sweden and The Netherlands). This is often cited in support of home confinement and less medical intervention in normal pregnancy, but multiple factors are involved in analysing the rate in any one setting.

The falling PNM is due to:
– improved general health and social conditions
– better maternity services
– improved prenatal detection of abnormalities (ultrasound, genetic developments, amniocentesis) ... at the expense of increasing TOP rates
– improved neonatal facilities
– lower parity

The *major causes of perinatal death* include:
1. *Congenital anomalies* (either stillbirth or neonatal death), e.g. NTD, cardiac lesions.
2. *Prematurity*.
3. *Anoxia/asphyxia*: intrauterine leading to stillbirth or growth retardation particularly, and events occuring at the birth.

Can PNM be reduced?
1. *Congenital anomalies*. Around 2% of all babies have a congenital anomaly and half of these are major. Improvements could be made by:
– prevention, e.g. genetic counselling and risk assessment, pre- and periconceptual folate supplements to reduce NTD risk, preconceptual advice (e.g. for diabetics)

- screening for affected fetuses, e.g. antenatal serum screening for NTD and chromosomal anomaly by AFP or triple test, nuchal fold scanning for trisomy 21 and cardiac lesions, fetal anomaly scanning in the second trimester
- screening for at-risk women (e.g. rubella screening and immunisation)
- avoid teratogens

2. *Prematurity*. To date, there has been poor achievement in this area as regards prevention. Most advances are through better care of the preterm infant and accurate pregnancy dating by ultrasound, reducing the incidence of inappropriately timed elective delivery.
   - cervical cerclage if *genuine* history but beware increased risk of septic abortion. True cervical incompetence is rare
   - early diagnosis and use of suppressants/tocolytics, e.g. salbutamol or ritodrine
   - there may be some merit in new predictive tests for at-risk women (e.g. fetal fibronectin), allowing pre-delivery transfer to specialist neonatal units, or steroids etc. to be given to improve fetal lung maturity
   - use of steroids to accelerate fetal lung maturity
   - improved neonatal facilities
   - use of artificial surfactant on SCBU
   - improved ventilation techniques

3. *Risk selection*:
   - role of specialist obstetrician
   - importance of booking visit
   - appropriate choice of place of delivery
   antenatal low-dose aspirin for pre-eclampsia/IUGR. Multicentre 'CLASP' trial reported no proven benefit, but there was a suggestion of improvement in the prevention of repeated very early-onset pre-eclampsia and aspirin continues to be used for this

4. *Management of labour and delivery*:
   - avoid sepsis
   - avoid prolonged labour
   - avoid difficult instrumental delivery
   - adequately trained and supervised staff
   - resuscitation facilities
   - role of fetal monitoring by CTG uncertain, but it has gained wide acceptance: only of real use with experienced interpretation and in conjunction with fetal acid-base status measurement.
   - anaesthetic expertise.

Risk factors for PNM The following factors are associated with an increased risk of PNM:

1. *Maternal factors*
   - age (over 35 or under 16)
   - primigravida or grand multipara
   - low socioeconomic class
   - extremes of maternal weight
   - short stature (under 152 cm)
   - smoking

　　　　　– drug/alcohol abuse
　　　　　– certain maternal diseases, e.g. diabetes, connective tissue disease, renal disease
　　　2. *Past obstetric history*
　　　　　– any form of recurrent pregnancy failure
　　　　　　a) miscarriage
　　　　　　b) SB/NND
　　　　　　c) IUGR
　　　　　– premature labour
　　　　　– fetal anomalies
　　　　　– LSCS
　　　　　– previous haemorrhage/APH
　　　3. *Complications arising in this pregnancy*
　　　　　– gestational diabetes
　　　　　– hypertension
　　　　　– anaemia
　　　　　– APH
　　　　　– preterm labour
　　　　　– malpresentation
　　　　　– polyhydramnios *or* oligohydramnios
　　　　　– IUGR
　　　　　– multiple pregnancy

◆ Stillbirth

The stillbirth rate is the number of infants born with no signs of life after 24 weeks gestation per 1000 total births. The 1998 rate in England, Wales and N. Ireland was 5.0/1000, the lowest ever.

Note: *A live birth is registered at any gestation when there are signs of life recorded at birth, but only babies born >24 weeks with no signs of life are registered as stilllborn – earlier births without signs of life are registered as a miscarriage.*

◆ Neonatal death

The neonatal death rate is the number of infant deaths before 28 days per 1000 live births (regardless of length of gestation). The 1998 rate was 3.8/1000 live births.

Deaths in the first week of life (0–6 completed days) are termed 'early' neonatal deaths.

◆ Preconception clinics

The concept of pre-pregnancy advice is becoming increasingly relevant, particularly with increased public awareness of health issues in general. The GP's surgery should provide the ideal setting for most women, advising about:
– smoking/drinking and dietary issues
– family history and relevant risks
– rubella status
– HIV screening and status

- BP/smear/breast examination
- avoidance of teratogenic drugs
- preconceptual folic acid supplements
- information about basic antenatal care and screening (e.g. serum sreening/scans)

Detailed referral is necessary for:
- diabetes
- hypertension or renal disease
- thromboembolic disorder or tendency
- previous cardiac history (rheumatic heart disease is now uncommon, but survivors of cardiac surgery in childhood are increasingly common)
- genetic disorders (genetic research is advancing so quickly that prenatal diagnosis options increase almost every week)
- previous obstetric history of relevance
- HIV-positive women

◆ Diagnosis of pregnancy

Gestation in weeks is given in brackets.
1. The *symptoms* of pregnancy are:
   - amenorrhoea
   - nausea
   - tiredness
   - breast soreness/tingling
   - urinary frequency
   - fetal movements
   - colostrum, galactorrhoea
   - uterine cramps
2. The *signs* are:
   - cervical softening
   - nipple pigmentation
   - enlarged uterus
        large egg (6–8 weeks)
        grapefruit (10 weeks)
   - uterus palpable above pubis (usually 12 weeks)
   - fetal heart heard (from 14 to 16 weeks with a sonicaid)
   - fetal parts felt
3. *Tests*:
   - urine test. Sensitive urine tests can detect β-subunit of HCG on the first day of the missed period
   - vaginal ultrasound scan can detect the gestation sac at 6 weeks and the fetal heart by 7 weeks
   - ultrasound can date the pregnancy from around 7 weeks with accuracy (by crown–rump length measurement)

◆ Early development

1. The blastocyst implants 7 days after fertilisation. It consists of an outer trophoblast layer (the future chorion), an inner cell mass and

between them a chorionic space. It becomes buried beneath the decidua by the action of the trophoblastic enzymes.

2. The inner cell mass forms an embryonic plate (the future fetus) and an amniotic cavity which expands to surround the fetus, except for the cord, and obliterates the chorionic space (like a balloon expanding inside a balloon). The membranes therefore consist of two layers (outer chorion and inner amnion).

3. As it grows, the conceptus forms a bump beneath the decidua which enlarges to fill the whole uterus by 12 weeks. The decidua overlying the conceptus fuses with that on the opposite side (hence salpingitis, i.e. ascending infection, cannot occur after 12 weeks of pregnancy because the tubes are effectively blocked off).

4. The part of the trophoblast that implants first becomes the placenta and develops villi. The fetal umbilical vessels (two arteries, one vein) end as capillaries in each villus: thus, the fetal circulation is closed.

5. The spiral arteries of the uterus circulate maternal blood into the intervillous spaces. The bleeding in a threatened miscarriage and in retroplacental haemorrhage involves maternal, not fetal, blood loss. Poor invasion of the spiral arterioles by the trophoblast is probably significant in determining the future development of IUGR and pre-eclampsia.

6. By 8 weeks organogenesis is complete and the fetus is a miniature human the size of a jelly baby.

◆ Physiology of pregnancy

Most physiological systems undergo changes in pregnancy; the most important features are:

1. Hormonal changes
   - the trophoblast produces HCG
   - the corpus luteum produces progesterone and relaxin
   - the placenta produces:
     a) HCG
     b) human placental lactogen (HPL)
     c) prolactin
     d) progesterone
     e) oestriol (in a conversion from cholesterol → pregnenolone → DHEAS (in fetal adrenal) → hydroxylated DHEAS (in fetal liver) → oestriol in the placenta. Oestriol is not essential to pregnancy (in placental sulphatase deficiency no oestriol can be produced but the pregnancy is normal, problems occurring due to prolonged pregnancy and failure to initiate labour)
     f) prostaglandins
     g) other placental proteins (which may prove useful in the future as markers of placental function, but not yet), e.g. pregnancy-associated plasma protein A (PAPP-A), placental protein S (PPS)

Progesterone causes:
- glandular development (decidua, breasts)
- decreased myometrial activity

- decreased smooth muscle tone of:
  a) stomach and colon (predisposing to reflux and constipation)
  b) ureters (predisposing to pyelonephritis and remaining dilated until 12 weeks postpartum)
  c) veins (predisposing to varicosity)

  All the above are exacerbated by the growing mass in the pelvis and abdomen as pregnancy advances. Venous dilatation and pooling, together with changes in the placental circulation, help to lower the diastolic blood pressure by aroud 10–20 mmHg in early pregnancy
- progesterone is also responsible for the dyspnoea of pregnancy, causing chronic hyperventilation and lowered maternal pCO_2 (hence easier transfer of fetal CO_2 to the mother)

Oestriol causes uterine growth (the uterus increases from 60 g to 1 kg) and softening of the ligaments of the pubic symphysis (increasing pelvic dimensions), lumbar spine (leading to postural and balance changes but predisposing to root pain) and ribs (splaying to allow room for the enlarging uterine fundus).

Cortisol causes gluconeogenesis but insulin levels also rise so fasting blood sugar actually falls.

2. Cardiovascular changes

- increased blood volume (30% by 30 weeks)
- increased cardiac output (30% by 12 weeks, therefore impaired cardiac function either causes a problem by 12 weeks gestation or may not be too significant. The third stage of labour is also a difficult time for impaired cardiac patients due to the sudden pre-load increase as the uterine musculature contracts and empties blood rapidly into the circulation)
- haemodilution
- oedema (increased permcability of vessels)
- increased postural hypotension

3. Changes in clotting factors and function

All major clotting factors increase in pregnancy, increasing the risk of DVT and PE, particularly as the gravid uterus exacerbates stasis in the lower limbs. Patients with connective tissue disease, known thrombophilias, or a past history of thrombosis may require (prophylactic) anticoagulation before and after delivery.

4. Changes in biochemical/lab values

- increased red cell mass ⎫
- increased plasma volume ⎬ Hb falls, MCV normal
- increased WBC
- platelets may fall or rise
- increased ESR
- plasma viscosity is normal
- decreased albumin
- increased alkaline phosphatase (made by the placenta)
- increased creatinine clearance, lower serum creatinine (increased GFR and increased plasma volume)

– glycosuria is common as the renal threshold for glucose falls, but *persistent* glycosuria must not be ignored

5. **Respiratory changes**
– chronic hyperventilation
– dyspnoea as uterus enlarges
– lower maternal pCO_2 (assists transfer of O_2 and CO_2 to/from fetus)

6. **Weight changes**
Weight gain of pregnancy is about 10 kg (0.5 kg per week for the last 20 weeks). This is due to:
– fat and fluid (5 kg)
– fetus (3.5 kg)
– placenta (1 kg)
– amniotic fluid (0.5 kg)

Metabolic rate is increased in pregnancy and goitre can occur, but the free thyroxine index is normal.

Measuring the booking weight is useful but recording weight gain throughout pregnancy is a poor indicator of fetal outcome.

◆ Dietary advice in pregnancy

Extreme starvation influences birth weight and PNM but otherwise the average Western diet provides sufficient calories, proteins, vitamins and minerals for normal singleton pregnancies. Smaller more frequent meals may reduce nausea and reflux.

1. *Iron* supplementation remains controversial but there is solid evidence that although the Hb level may remain satisfactory, body stores of Fe are almost exhausted by term. Hb fall is the last indicator of Fe deficiency (measure serum ferritin if there is any doubt). Routine Fe prophylaxis for all pregnant women is advisable unless there is specific intolerance. In multiple pregnancy Fe and folate supplementation is *essential*.
Typical preparations provide 100 mg Fe + 500 μg folic acid, e.g.
   – Pregaday (ferrous fumarate 304 mg + folic acid 350 μg)
   – Ferrograd Folic (slow release ferrous sulphate 325 mg + folic acid 350 μg)

2. *Folic acid*. There is evidence that prophylaxis (400 μg daily) before and in the first 12 weeks of pregnancy reduces the risk of NTD. The Chief Medical Officer and RCOG Advisory Committee recommend folic acid supplementation for all women to reduce risk of NTD.

3. *B12*. No evidence for requirement of supplementation.

4. *Vitamin D*. Supplementation may be indicated in Asian mothers, or in those with past history of rickets (dose = 400 U/day throughout pregnancy).

5. *Calcium* supplements are popular for lactating women but there is little scientific evidence of benefit.

6. *Specific foods*. Pregnant women should avoid:
   – excessive vitamin A (liver) – teratogenesis
   – unpasteurised cheese – *Listeria*
   – raw eggs, undercooked meats – *Salmonella* and toxoplasmosis

◆ Alcohol, smoking and drug-taking in pregnancy

1. *Alcohol.* Heavy drinking is associated with teratogenesis, cardiac anomalies and later, severe IUGR. Fetal alcohol syndrome (growth retardation, dysmorphic features, mental retardation) is rare but catastrophic.

   Moderate alcohol consumption (1–2 units/day) may be associated with minor anomalies but the data are inconclusive.

2. *Smoking.* Heavy smoking (>25 cigarettes/day) causes reduced birth weight (by 150–250 g at term) due to placental vasoconstriction effects. Also:
   - thrombotic risks are increased
   - the CTG may be unreactive for up to 1 hour after cigarettes (reflecting presumed decrease in O_2 transfer to fetus)
   - pre-eclampsia is slightly less common in smokers (reasons unclear)
   - smoking by any of the family at home is associated with increased risk of cot death (SIDS)

3. *Drugs.* Addictive drugs (heroin, methadone, cocaine) cause growth retardation, withdrawal symptoms and sedation in the neonate.

◆ Antenatal care

Different models of antenatal care exist, but in the UK they all follow a similar pattern, with care being given by:
- consultant only
- shared care (consultant/GP/midwife)
- GP unit (GP/midwife), or
- midwife only

Supporting lay groups (National Childbirth Trust, Laleche, etc.) provide valuable classes, booklets and advice.

Booking visit Most women present to the GP at 8–10 weeks of pregnancy. The GP should:
- confirm pregnancy (β-HCG if doubt)
- define risk factors and refer appropriately
- discuss antenatal care and place of delivery

Important aspects of the history include:
- age, parity, ? planned pregnancy
- smoking, drugs (HIV status), alcohol
- previous history   – infertility
  - pregnancy/delivery events
  - medical problems, previous surgery
- present pregnancy – bleeding?/pain?
  - excessive symptoms, e.g. nausea
  - movements (usually > 16–20 weeks)
- LMP (regular?, previous O/C pill?, certain?)
- social factors (single?, partner?, access to appropriate information and supporting agencies)
- family history   – congenital anomaly
  - ethnic features? (e.g. for haemoglobinopathies)

- diabetes?
- hypertension?

Examination
- uterine size, dates? (PV)
- height/weight/shoe size
- BP
- urinalysis
- smear?, HVS?
- chest, heart, breasts
- fetal heart sounds?

The accurate assessment of gestation is the cornerstone of antenatal management. Early ultrasound is more reliable than a certain LMP at predicting EDD but clinicians rarely change dates if scan and LMP dates are within 1 week of one another. Only 5% of babies arrive on the EDD. PNM is lowest between 38 and 42 weeks.

Most consultant delivery units provide guidelines as to who is and is not suitable for GP care. (Know your local guidelines as an example.)

Pregnancy progress
Fundal height (with an empty bladder)
- palpable over symphysis (12 weeks)
- umbilicus (22 weeks)
- xiphisternum (36 weeks)

Measure height in cm from symphysis to fundus (S–F height in cm = number of weeks, from 16 to 36 weeks) as well as in finger breadths. More than 3 cm discrepancy in dates is significant.

Small for dates:
- wrong dates/transverse lie
- IUGR (if severe, check FH? fetal death in utero)
- oligohydramnios
- fetal anomaly, especially chromosomal

Large for dates:
- wrong dates
- multiple pregnancy
- polyhydramnios
- hydatidiform mole
- large baby (?diabetes)
- fetal anomaly (especially hydrocephalus, NTD)

Routine antenatal checks
Note: Mothers should be counselled carefully about what each test is for and give consent for any investigation (especially for Down's syndrome screening), any ultrasound scans and for HIV screening (which is now widely advocated). It is vital that the implications of any possible result are clear *before* performing the test.

The majority of care will be provided by the primary care team, referring to hospital specialists only if necessary.
1. Initial booking (preferably by 10 weeks)
   - Hb (haemoglobinopathy if relevant)
   - group and antibodies (Rhesus and atypical)
   - rubella antibodies (immunise postpartum if negative)

- VDRL (FTA/TPI if any doubt)
- HIV status (if *fully* counselled)
2. At 15–18 weeks
   - AFP sometimes (but detailed USS is more reliable for detection of NTD)
   - ±serum screening for Down's syndrome (often known as the 'triple' or 'double' test). These tests use a combination of the individual woman's details such as age, weight, ethnic group, smoking history and her levels of AFP/HCG/oestriol (expressed as multiples of the median or MOMs), to predict the risk of Down's syndrome. Scan dating is considered essential to allow an accurate assessment of the risk. The result is expressed as 'high' or 'low' risk, with or without a *specific* risk quoted, depending on the lab used. Women at high risk may wish to have an amniocentesis. (See section on prenatal testing)

   (**Note**: *these tests are not available in all districts, but you must be familiar with at least one scheme for the exam.*)
   Hospital booking varies: if required, it is at 9–20 weeks, depending on your local arrangements, and often will be linked to a dating scan or structural scan appointment. Many units use a system of mothers carrying their own notes which lessens the risk of lost results/notes and is popular with mothers.
3. From 18–20 weeks to delivery, appointments will be:
   - monthly to 28 weeks
   - fortnightly to 36 weeks
   - weekly to 40 weeks or delivery

What to look for **Note**: There is no ideal time to pick up a specific complication such as IUGR or pre-eclampsia but signs become more obvious from 28–32 weeks onwards. Remain vigilant in every case.
1. *Weight gain* – the least important of all antenatal clinical signs but weight *loss* is significant.
   Normal range is 10–12 kg overall
   Normal range is 0.5 kg/week (20–40 weeks)
   Excessive weight gain may indicate oedema
2. *BP*
   - often drops slightly in second trimester, rising to original level in third trimester
   - should be measured consistently in semi-upright position with appropriate size cuff for arm dimensions. Poor measurement leads to unnecessary intervention. (A second elevated level after a 20-minute interval is significant.)
3. *Urinalysis*
   - trace glycosuria is common. Ask for a second fasting specimen to test
   - trace proteinuria could indicate contaminated sample (repeat and send MSU) or infection. '+' or more is significant and demands investigation. 24-hour collections of <0.3 g usually register as trace or '+' on dipstick. More than 0.3 g/24 hours is *always* abnormal.
   - *Proteinuria should never be dismissed lightly.*

◆ Prenatal screening and diagnostic tests

Many conditions are now amenable to prenatal diagnosis and genetic advances occur daily – refer for up-to-date information to a specialist centre.

Screening tests are either:
- general population screen offered to all, e.g. AFP at 16 weeks
- specific screening tests in a high-risk group, e.g. glucose load or GTT if family history, etc.

Screening is a form of risk assessment; definitive diagnosis requires further specific tests if the screen shows positive results, e.g. high-resolution ultrasound if AFP increased, amniocentesis if triple test screen positive/higher than expected.

Counselling is a vital part of screening and the consequences of positive and negative screening tests should be fully discussed *before* doing the screening test. The timing (gestation) of individual screening tests is usually critical (hence value of dating USS early on).

Serum screening tests

For NTD:
- blood test at 16 weeks. High levels in the fetus cause elevations in maternal serum AFP where feto-maternal barriers are breached, e.g.
    open spina bifida
    abdominal wall defects
    anencephaly
    fetal death
    bleeding in pregnancy
- result expressed as multiple of the median for gestation (MOM): usually >2.2 MOM is considered raised and further investigation warranted. (Repeat level and detailed USS. Amniocentesis for AFP and acetylcholinesterase levels in liquor has been largely superseded by detailed USS but may still have some role in difficult cases.)

For chromosomal anomaly:
The triple test (sometimes called 'Bart's' test as devised by Cuckle and Wald at St Bartholomew's Hospital); also the similar Leeds test (where four hormonal parameters are assessed). These are screening tests for assessing the risk of trisomy 21 but other patterns in the result may suggest T 18 or other chromosomal defects, or pick up fetal demise in utero. They are unhelpful in multiple pregnancy, and in diabetics accuracy is improved by using a different reference range.
- maternal blood
- 15+ to 18 weeks
- AFP, oestriol and HCG levels interpreted as MOM. Bart's test classes absolute risk$>1:250$ as screen positive. Maternal age, gestation, weight, ethnic origin also used in the assessment of an individual pregnancy risk. Mothers perceived to be at high risk may want to progress to amniocentesis as the *diagnostic* test

Reports where risk is compared with that expected due to age alone are not always helpful. Comparing the more sensitive and specific serum result with a known inferior test (age alone) may lead to inappropriate anxiety: for example, a risk of 1 : 1000 is still low relative to the risk of miscarriage from a diagnostic procedure, even if the risk based on age alone was 1 : 2000. Conversely, false reassurance may be taken from a relative reduction in risk from 1 : 50 based on age alone, to 1 : 80 from serum screening. *Both* these risks are greater than the risk of pregnancy loss from amniocentesis. Clearly, careful pre-test counselling is vital and everyone involved in antenatal care must be absolutely clear about this type of screening.

In older mothers, their age weights the result, so a high proportion of results come back with a 'high' risk. However, the false negative rate is low, so 'low'-risk results are more likely to be true negatives. This makes the test useful in helping older mothers avoid amniocentesis, which many of them may wish to do if their experience involves previous pregnancy loss, infertility or a late start to childbearing.

Conversely, the test may be of less use in very young mothers and for this reason, some districts will not offer it below a certain age on cost-effective grounds. Serum screening of this type does have greater predictive value than maternal age alone but still has sensitivity of only 60–70%. There is much misunderstanding about use of the triple test and counselling should be improved considerably.

Cystic fibrosis screening

– birth prevalance 1 : 2500
– CF is the commonest autosomal recessive condition in the UK. One in 25 adults are carriers (2×10^6 asymptomatic carriers in the UK). The gene is carried on the long arm of chromosome 7
– recent genetic advances have identified genetic markers (deletions) accounting for the majority of cases ($\triangle$F508 accounts for 75%, G551D accounts for a further 5%)

'Couple screening' is simple (mouthwash samples from male and female partners, analysing second sample only if first test is positive), cheap and identifies *couples* at risk of having an affected fetus. Amniocentesis can identify the gene deletion. However, screening *in a pregnancy* is not ideal as it involves later diagnostic tests if there are delays. Pre-pregnancy screening will be valueless if there is uncertainty about paternity.

Note: Some affected fetuses without the commonest gene deletions will be missed.

Pre-implantation genetic diagnosis

May offer useful help for couples with high genetic risks if the involved gene has been identified, and has already been sucessfully used in Tay-Sachs carriers.

Ultrasound screening

2% of babies have a congenital anomaly, mainly structural defects, and half of these will be considered to be severe. Many such structural defects can be detected on detailed USS, but many minor ones will be missed. Some trisomies (especially trisomy 13 and trisomy 18) commonly have structural anomalies ('markers') but amniocentesis for chromosome analysis will still be required for confirmation. Approximately 50% of Down's syndrome fetuses will show a significant structural defect, especially cardiac anomaly, but even so-called 'soft markers' may be absent and trisomy 21 cannot be reliably detected on USS.

Many districts offer anomaly scanning as a routine: acceptance is almost 100%.

Ideally, structural scans are performed at 19–20 weeks gestation, as earlier timing may miss cardiac or renal anomalies, and the oligohydramnios associated with renal anomaly may not be evident before fetal urine production begins to have a significant effect on the liquor volume. Other anomalies such as diaphragmatic hernia may, however, not be evident even at this stage. Diagnosis is more difficult in the obese and these women are best scanned a little later. Most NTDs can be seen earlier so elevated maternal sAFP or prior history may make a first look at 16 weeks worthwhile.

Accuracy depends on:
– high resolution equipment
– operator expertise
– methodical examination and reference to standard measurements
– fetal position
– maternal obesity

Organs usually checked are:
1. Head and neck
    – integrity of cranial vault
    – shape of the head (e.g. classical lemon/banana sign in NTD)
    – cerebellum
    – ventricles
    – nuchal thickness (see below)
    – cystic hygroma (may indicate Turner's syndrome)
2. Spine
3. Heart
    – 4 chamber view
    – major vessel connections/outflow tracts
    – rate and rhythm
4. Anterior abdominal wall (gastroschisis/exomphalos)
5. Stomach
6. Bladder
7. Kidneys
8. Limbs, hands and feet (talipes, chromosome anomaly)
9. Face
    – lip
    – palate
10. Liquor volume
11. Placental site and cord vessels

A single abnormal finding demands a detailed search for others. Second opinion referral if suspect.

Nuchal fold scanning is increasingly accepted as a valid screening test and may well be the best test for Down's syndrome. The sensitivity and specificity equal or exceed those achieved by serum screening in experienced centres. Other trisomies and major cardiac anomalies may also be suspected in this way. Nuchal translucency is of particular value in multiple pregnancy as each fetus can be assessed individually.

Invasive fetal diagnostic/therapeutic procedures

Almost all use *ultrasound-guided* techniques. These may involve:
- chromosome count and structure
- gene probe technology
- metabolic assays

Amniocentesis
- usually at 15–17 weeks for karyotyping, results in 2–3 weeks as fetal cells need time to grow in culture prior to counting chromosomes (can be done earlier but uncertain long-term risks)
- 10 ml liquor required for chromosomes/AFP and acetylcholinesterase
- 0.5–1% miscarriage risk
- potential risk of fetal injury
- longer term risks include preterm labour or R/M
- can be done for multiple pregnancies if dye used to identify separate sacs
- also use in later pregnancy for Hb, haematocrit, genotype and bilirubin assay in Rhesus-affected fetus
- as indicated for metabolic or genetic studies
- rapid result in 24–48 hours using 'FISH' technique (fluorescent in-situ hybridisation) if looking for a particular chromosome with a known probe, e.g. a suspected trisomy found on USS

Chorionic villus sampling (CVS)
- needle sample/aspiration/biopsy of chorionic villi
- 10–12 weeks (< 10 weeks associated with limb reduction defects in recent series)
- transabdominal route favoured (less infection compared with transcervical)
- higher miscarriage rate (2–3%), therefore reserve for higher risk cases (e.g. autosomal recessive 1 : 4 risks)
- problems with mosaicism may lead to confusing result

Cordocentesis
- fetal blood obtained via umbilical vein in cord (or fetal intrahepatic portion of umbilical vein)
- usually in later pregnancy for diagnostic/therapeutic reasons (e.g. in-utero transfusions)
- increased miscarriage/preterm labour risk but fetuses already at high risk in this group
- fetal bradycardia a risk (especially if umbilical artery breached)

Fetoscopy
Visual inspection of fetus in utero using an endoscope. May rarely be useful but USS-guided techniques more common.

Notes
1. Discuss options with local genetic specialist centre when choosing which test is appropriate.
2. Give anti-D to Rhesus-negative mothers to prevent iso-immunisation.
3. USS has revolutionised prenatal diagnosis and therapy.

◆ Fetal surveillance

Assessment of the fetus includes attention to growth, development and behaviour patterns (movements and heart rate, etc.).

'Monitoring' is most useful from 26 weeks (i.e. from the time the fetus is normally viable) in conditions associated with acute intrauterine compromise, but is a poor predictor of future fetal wellbeing. It can cause increased anxiety and apart from allowing planned preemptive delivery, does not affect any therapeutic decisions.

Fetal activity charts

Reduction in movements *may* indicate an 'ill' fetus but large-scale trials on 'kick charts' have proved less helpful than at first thought. Maternal observations, however, remain a vital part of detecting changes in fetal activity levels and should never be ignored.

In one method (the kick chart) the woman notes the time each day by when she has counted 10 fetal movements (not just 'kicks') starting at 9 am. However, some women don't notice fetal movements and others may become over-anxious using this method.

If the woman has felt no movements for 12 hours or notices a change in pattern, she should attend for a cardiotocograph.

Cardiotocography

The CTG is a continuous recording of the fetal heart rate and rhythm (using external ultrasound) and of maternal contractions (using a tocometer).

The frequency of CTG tracing is dictated by the circumstances. A normal CTG does not predict future safety for the fetus over any defined period of time – it is an assessment of the *current* position. It is performed for 20–40 minutes and gives an indication of current fetal well-being. A normal trace is reassuring but needs to be interpreted in the context of the rest of the pregnancy assessment.

A flat trace (poor beat-to-beat variation) with no accelerations in heart rate on fetal movement (non-reactive trace) may suggest chronic hypoxia, but the tracing should be continued over a longer period as the mature fetus has defined sleep/activity cycles, with the 'sleep' pattern rarely exceeding 45 minutes. Chronic hypoxia is more reliably detected by using serial (computerised) analysis of CTGs than by the naked eye. Computerised CTG assessment takes gestation into account and if normal parameters are met swiftly, the trace may be discontinued. This reduces the time spent on monitoring and is cost-effective for staff and mothers.

Experience in detecting trends in CTG changes (less variation, higher baseline rate, small decelerations) is vital. If other tests are also poor (few movements, poor growth rate) delivery may be considered.

A very poor trace (e.g. fetal tachycardia, poor short-term variability and unprovoked decelerations) can be an indication for emergency caesarean section.

Monitoring is most used for chronic conditions which are associated with changes in placental function (IUGR, diabetes, hypertension, Rhesus disease, multiple pregnancy, APH) and for situations which may compromise the fetus acutely such as haemorrhage or abruption.

Biochemical tests of placental function

Research into newer biochemical markers (e.g. PAPP-A) continues. They have no certain role as yet. Previous tests (oestriol, HPL) are of no clinical value.

Ultrasound monitoring

- fetal growth
- fetal activity
- liquor volume (reduced in IUGR)
- Doppler flow studies on placental/fetal vessels/cord

Serial *growth estimations* are the most useful. HC/AC should be plotted graphically (highlighting asymmetrical IUGR). Other parameters such as BPD and femur length are less closely linked with growth assessment. AC is largely determined by liver size and will indicate a well-nourished fetus. The 'brain-sparing' effect of IUGR allows nourishment to go to the most important organs – the head, heart and lungs.

In *biophysical profile assessment* movements, tone, fetal breathing activity, liquor volume and CTG are observed and scored in a reproducible way. The equal scoring weight of each parameter, however, obscures the fact that severely reduced liquor is of much more significance than, say, fetal breathing.

Specialised *'Doppler' flow studies* may suggest compromised flow in the placental circulation/umbilical cord (end-diastolic flow reduced, absent or reversed in a high-resistance placental circuit). These studies may also pick up differential flow between fetal carotids/middle cerebral arteries and the descending aorta, implying shunting of blood to the brain in asymmetrical IUGR. The significance for low-risk women can be misleading, however, with poor sensitivity and specificity.

Most hospitals now have an 'Assessment Unit' where at-risk mothers can be supervised on an outpatient basis. This has proved extremely cost-effective in terms of reducing admissions for 'rest and assessment' for fetal movements, hypertension, diabetes, etc. There is no evidence that routine fetal assessment in the third trimester in low-risk mothers improves outcome.

Some units routinely monitor post-term pregnancies by CTG/biophysical profile assessment but there is little evidence of benefit unless dates are uncertain. It can be useful if mothers wish to avoid induction of labour (after, e.g. 42 weeks) but sudden intrauterine death can occur despite apparently normal surveillance results at *any* gestation.

The HC increases by about 3 mm per week from 20 weeks and by 1 mm per week at term. At least a fortnight is needed between scans to monitor growth rate reliably. One set of measurements on a fetus is of little help because size obviously varies between individuals, unless the situation is extreme.

Notes

1. These tests are used together as a guide to the condition of the fetus. It is the *overall pattern* that dictates management. Ask yourself if the fetus is better off 'in' or 'out'. The gestation and SCBU facilities available are important in making your decision.
2. Changes in fetal well-being are detected over different timescales by different methods.
   - CTG (hours)
   - kick chart (hours)
   - scans (weeks)

◆ Intrauterine growth retardation

Perinatal mortality and morbidity is increased in growth-restricted fetuses due to chronic intrauterine hypoxia, intrapartum hypoxia and acidosis. The cause may be fetal, maternal or joint. IUGR is one of the commonest factors in perinatal deaths (with congenital abnormality and prematurity).

Definition of IUGR varies but < 10th centile for gestation is a common working approach. However, the fetuses most at risk are those below the 3rd centile, and those whose growth falls well below their expected pattern ('relative IUGR').

Features suggesting placental insufficiency are:
1. Poor maternal weight gain, when sustained as < 0.5 kg/week for several weeks. Note that excessive weight gain due to pre-eclampsia may also conceal IUGR.
2. Clinically small-for-dates. The fundal height in cm above the symphysis pubis should be within 3 cm of the gestation in weeks. In addition there may be oligohydramnios. Refer to confirm or refute the diagnosis of IUGR by USS, check the gestation, exclude fetal abnormality and monitor the fetus if IUGR confirmed.

   Clinical examination alone misses over 40% IUGR. Ultrasound improves this considerably but single measurements are of little value. Research suggests that the use of 'customised' growth charts taking account of an individual's ethnic group, height, weight, POH and other factors may improve detection rate. Standardised charts of fetal growth are available and serial plotting of measurements is extremely useful.
3. Reduced fetal movement is usually unhelpful at spotting IUGR in an otherwise low-risk case, but should prompt proper assessment.

Risk factors   Major risk factors for IUGR are:
   – previous history (2.9 kg at term is approx. 10th centile)
   – pre-eclampsia
   – smoking/alcohol
   – APH
   – multiple pregnancy
   – fetal abnormality
   – extremes of maternal height/weight and age
   – maternal renal disease
   – maternal diabetes (although these fetuses are more often large)
   – other maternal disease
      connective tissue disorder (SLE)
      autoimmune disease (antiphospholipid syndrome)
      thrombophilia (Factor V Leiden mutation)
      haemoglobinopathies (rarely)
      untreated hyperthyroidism
      severe chronic lung/heart disease (rarely)
   – severe malnutrition

Management   – confirm the dates (to exclude incorrect maturity)
   – refer to assess the fetus
   – look for a cause (commonly pre-eclampsia)

- deliver in a unit with SCBU (in-utero transfer if needed)
- consider steroid prophylaxis for fetal lung maturity
- postpone delivery as long as the fetal condition is satisfactory, then decide best mode of delivery
- continuous fetal monitoring in labour
- epidural is the preferred analgesia for labour or C/S: avoids opiates
- short controlled second stage is indicated for vaginal delivery
- suck out any meconium from the pharynx at birth and monitor blood sugars for 72 hours by Dextrostix. Frequent feeds

The baby's weight will be below the 10th centile for its gestational age, and such a light-for-dates (dysmature) infant has fourfold increase in neonatal death rate from:
- meconium aspiration
- hypoglycaemia
- hypothermia

◆ Pre-eclampsia (PET)

Classically, a syndrome of:
- marked oedema
- hypertension (traditionally above 140/90 mmHg, but more realistically above 170/110 mmHg in late pregnancy, and then considered an obstetric emergency)
- proteinuria (above 0.3 g/l per 24 hours)

Now, however, thought of much more as a true multi-system disease, probably one end of a spectrum of conditions including IUGR, PET with fetal compromise/IUGR, and purely 'maternal' PET with a well-grown fetus.

Pre-eclampsia rarely occurs before 28 weeks and is seen in 5–10% of pregnancies. The patient is usually primigravid and it is more likely to develop in the very young or in the older mother. The incidence rises if there is already hypertension, renal or connective tissue disease, and in multiple pregnancy. The recurrence risk is about 15% – usually less severe and later in onset – and rises with a new partner. Much earlier onset can occur in molar pregnancy and in some fetal trisomies, especially Edwards' syndrome (T 18).

Both perinatal and maternal mortality and morbidity are increased.

Clinical sequelae
1. *Risks to mother*
   - cerebrovascular accident (haemorrhage)
   - eclamptic fits
   - renal/liver failure
   - abruption
   - coagulopathy (disseminated intravascular coagulation)
   - HELLP syndrome (haemolysis, elevated liver enzymes, low platelets)
   - iatrogenic (e.g. fluid overload, operative delivery)
2. *Risks to fetus*
   - IUGR (and sequelae)
   - fetal death in utero (growth failure or APH)
   - extreme prematurity and its sequelae

Pre-eclampsia is thought to be caused by an immunologically mediated failure of secondary placentation with defective invasion and dilatation of maternal spiral arterioles by the trophoblast. Vasoactive substances emanating from the placenta may play a part in the later presentation of the disease. Pathophysiology suggests predetermination, probably before 20 weeks, leading to optimism that the condition may be detected by Doppler flow studies of the uteroplacental circulation. This would allow concentration of resources towards those at risk but, so far, screening low-risk populations has proved unhelpful. Known high-risk groups are currently offered close surveillance anyway, so early prediction would offer little additional benefit.

Assessment   The key to good management is *early detection*. Oedema is the least important sign. It is generalised (pretibial, face, fingers) and causes excessive weight gain (1 kg/week). With marked oedema, increase the frequency of antenatal visits to monitor the BP. Diuretics aggravate intravascular volume depletion, do not alter the course of PET and should be avoided.

Refer for investigation if *hypertension* develops (sustained BP above 140/90) or if there is a rise in diastolic pressure of more than 15 mmHg above the booking level. Rest may lower the BP and improve placental blood flow but is unlikely to be useful if the placental circulation is compromised and risks increasing the tendency to thrombosis. Outpatient investigation at a day unit is almost always preferred, but proteinuric women *must* be admitted as the situation is more likely to be genuine and may advance rapidly (in hours).

Exclude other causes of hypertension (MSU, U&E, possibly 24-hour VMA), assess the severity and monitor the situation. Admission can be helpful to assess the night-time BP profile (rises in pre-eclampsia, falls in the normal) and:
- 4-hourly BP
- 24-hour protein excretion
- creatinine clearance
- serial uric acid levels (may rise)
- serial platelet counts (may fall)
- liver function (transaminases – AST, ALT and bilirubin)

Assess fetal well-being (see above).

In hypertension without significant 'pre-eclampsia', the BP usually settles quickly and the woman can be reviewed regularly in the antenatal clinic by the GP or community midwife. Fetal surveillance should continue. These cases rarely run into more serious trouble.

Admission is indicated if:
- BP rises steadily. Urgent if above 170/110 mmHg.
- proteinuria develops (a sign that PET is progressive. If proteinuria develops, inpatient monitoring is essential as condition can deteriorate rapidly)
- there is evidence of IUGR or fetal compromise
- any symptoms develop

Note: Pre-eclampsia is usually asymptomatic right up until the late stages of the condition. First presentation may be with eclampsia.

Management of pre-eclampsia:
- maternal monitoring (weight, BP, proteinuria)
- monitor the fetus
- group and save serum (emergency section)
- watch platelet count, AST/ALT, haematocrit, urine volumes

Antihypertensives may be appropriate in specialist centres, but only to protect the mother or to advance the gestation under close surveillance. A sustained maternal BP of > 170/110 mmHg must be treated urgently (e.g. nifedipine 10 mg stat) to reduce the risk of cerebral haemorrhage – a significant cause of maternal death from pre-eclampsia.

Delivery:
- planned, usually at term
- sooner if significant maternal/fetal compromise
- vaginal route if favourable

Pre-eclampsia resolves after delivery. The definitive treatment for severe pre-eclampsia remains urgent delivery. After delivery the condition usually resolves rapidly although during the first 48 hours it may deteriorate or be unstable. The majority of eclampsia still occurs *after* delivery: remain vigilant, especially with regard to fluid balance. Short-term complications may require ITU help; long-term sequelae are very rare.

Fulminating pre-eclampsia and eclampsia
- assess the severity: check for symptoms of pre-eclampsia (headache, nausea, vomiting, epigastric pain, blurred vision, 'jitters') and signs (photophobia, hyper-reflexia and clonus, epigastric (liver) tenderness, confusion and restlessness)
- assess the fetus
- multidisciplinary approach
- deliver

Management
- antihypertensive agents (aim for diastolic of 90–100 mmHg)
- anticonvulsants? (debated, current multicentre trial on benefit in severe PET and eclampsia)
- review liver/renal function/albumin/coagulation
- extremely close watch on fluid balance vital (leaky capillaries → pulmonary and cerebral oedema). Fluid overload is a common problem

Vaginal delivery preferable, but caesarean section is often appropriate. Regional anaesthesia is not contraindicated if platelet count is > 100 000.

Under 34 weeks emergency section is usually performed because induction is difficult and fetal distress more likely.

Antihypertensive medication saves lives:
- BP of 170/110 mmHg is an obstetric emergency
- Use hydralazine/nifedipine/labetalol stat and to follow
- deliver when BP controlled (intubation causes significant increase in systolic BP)

Anti-convulsant medication is indicated to *control* a fit ($MgSO_4$ or Diazemuls). There is uncertainty about the benefit of prophylaxis – most units use magnesium.

Magnesium sulphate: No agent is proven to prevent recurrence of fits, but magnesium sulphate is preferred. It is safe, the mother stays alert, it is relatively effective at preventing future fits, is also antihypertensive, and requires reasonably simple monitoring. (The main risk is of respiratory suppression, without sedation.) A typical regimen is a 4 g loading dose i.v. slowly, then infusion of 1–2 g/hour. Continue for 24 hours after the last fit or until the investigations show improvement. Deep tendon reflexes are lost at moderate doses, large doses depress respiration and cause cardiac and respiratory arrest – monitor oxygen saturation, reflexes, serum Mg and creatinine levels and urine output. Excretion is via the kidney – adjust the regimen if there is oliguria. The specific antidote is calcium gluconate. Mg does not sedate the mother or fetus.

The risks of the alternatives (used widely before magnesium gained popularity) are: respiratory suppression, inhalation of vomit, fluid overload; and sedation of the mother and baby (esp. *diazepam*). Heminevrin (*chlormethiazole*) causes heavy sedation and is a poor anticonvulsant. It also requires administration of a large fluid volume, which is contraindicated. *Phenytoin* has been used in some centres and requires monitoring of the ECG and the K$^+$. None of them prevents further fits.

Prevention of pre-eclampsia

Low-dose aspirin (75 mg daily) may be of benefit in reducing pre-eclampsia as it reduces platelet coagulation to capillary walls (thought to be factor in aetiology). CLASP (Collaborative Low Dose Aspirin in Pregnancy) reported in 1994 on its use in double-blind placebo-controlled trial in many thousands of women. Despite encouraging subgroup results suggesting benefit in reducing pre-eclampsia, *none* of the results was substantially significant. However, the safety of aspirin use was proven conclusively; in particular, there was no increase in haemorrhage risk.

◆ Pre-existing (essential) hypertension

The BP falls in pregnancy, especially in the middle trimester (the systolic by about 10 mmHg and the diastolic by about 20 mmHg) due to vasodilation and the low resistance of the placental circulation. Women already on medication can often stop it in early pregnancy, restarting when required, usually not before 20–24 weeks.

BP above 140/90 in the first 24 weeks of pregnancy implies the existence of hypertension *before* pregnancy and occurs in about 1%. About 30% of such women develop pre-eclampsia (a further rise in BP with oedema and proteinuria).

BP above 170/100 increases the fetal loss to 30% due to accelerated placental degeneration and an increased risk of placental abruption. The maternal risks are LVF or cerebral haemorrhage.

Assessment

Any *cause* for the hypertension must be excluded:
– renal disease (MSU, U&E, creatinine clearance)
– renal artery stenosis (abdominal systolic bruit)
– coarctation (decreased and delayed femoral pulses)

- phaeochromocytoma (24-hour urinary VMA – rare)
- hydatidiform mole (ultrasound scan)

and the duration assessed:
- fundi (A–V nipping, haemorrhages, exudates, papilloedema)
- LVH (apex beat, CXR, ECG)

Management
- *bedrest* and monitor the BP. Often this is enough to control the BP, particularly as it falls in the middle trimester.

If not:
- *methyldopa* (initially 250 mg t.d.s.) is known to be safe and effective in pregnancy and does not adversely affect fetal growth. Aim for a diastolic of 90 mmHg (maternal *hypotension* can cause fetal death). *This does not prevent pre-eclampsia from developing.* β-blockers have been used widely but may cause impaired fetal growth, heart rate monitoring difficulties and neonatal hypoglycaemia. Good control of hypertension reduces PNM and decreases intervention, e.g. fewer preterm deliveries
- monitor the fetus. Serial scans (IUGR suggests superimposed pre-eclampsia). Induce at 38 weeks or earlier if the fetal condition is deteriorating. Section is often performed if delivery is necessary before 36 weeks
- serial maternal biochemistry tests: treating the BP masks impending pre-eclampsia
- *lifelong follow-up* is necessary

◆ Diabetes

Diabetes is associated with an increased PNM due to an increased incidence of:
- congenital abnormalities ($\times 4$)
- intrauterine death (? cause)
- long labour (large baby), trauma at birth (maternal and fetal)
- RDS
- IUGR
- prematurity (iatrogenic)

With good control there should be no increase in the incidence of a big baby, hydramnios, pre-eclampsia or UTI. Clinically there are two distinct situations:
1. Impaired glucose tolerance in pregnancy
2. Pregnancy in a known diabetic

Gestational impaired glucose tolerance
This is symptomless but increases the PNM to around 50 per 1000. It is suspected if there are any potential diabetic features:
- glycosuria ($\times 1$ before 20 weeks; $\times 2$ (10% will have an abnormal GTT) after 20 weeks)
- obesity
- FH of diabetes (in first-degree relative)
- previous gestational diabetes
- previous big baby (10 lb or 4.5 kg at term)
- previous unexplained PNM

- RDS or hypoglycaemia in previous babies
- hydramnios

Note: Glycosuria in *early* pregnancy is more likely to be due to diabetes than threshold changes. Test an early morning specimen to avoid postprandial glycosuria.

However, 30% of patients with gestational glucose intolerance do *not* have these features. A 'glucose load' test is therefore sometimes advocated at 16 and 28 weeks to screen women at higher risk. Most units do GLT only in at-risk groups (see above): a 50 g glucose drink is taken (non-fasting) and a blood test taken 1 hour later. Levels above 7.5 mmol/l (although this depends on the lab) indicate the need for a full GTT.

At a consensus conference in 1996 the 'St Vincent Task Force' agreed on the following:

Screening:
- test urine for glycosuria at every visit
- do timed random lab blood glucose measurements as follows
    whenever glycosuria > + is noted
    at the booking visit and at 28 weeks
- do a 75 g oral GTT if the timed random glucose is
    > 6 mmol/l when fasting or 2 hours after food
    > 7 mmol/l within 2 hours of food

Diagnosis: by 75 g oral GTT, according to revised WHO criteria (see Table 5).

Table 5   Range of glucose levels in 75 g glucose tolerance test (WHO)

	Fasting glucose level	*2-hour glucose level*
normal	<6 mmol/l	<9 mmol/l
gestational IGT	6–8 mmol/l	9–11 mmol/l
diabetes	>8 mmol/l	>11 mmol/l

Note: The blood glucose levels in pregnancy should be normal – fasting glucose is a bit lower and the peak after glucose a bit higher.

Management
- referral to specialist obstetric/diabetic clinic, if available
- blood sugar series on a normal diet. Preprandial glucose estimations throughout one day. If the average exceeds 5.5 mmol/l, treatment is indicated
- 150 g carbohydrate diet with high fibre. Repeat blood sugar series. If still above 5.5 mmol/l, insulin is indicated
- human short- and intermediate-acting insulin is started and blood glucose monitored. If glucose peaks occur a q.d.s regimen with Actrapid can be useful
- fetal surveillance (see above)
- there is no good evidence to support delivery before term in patients not requiring insulin and without complications, and after 40 weeks the same applies
- patients needing insulin are managed at delivery as for pre-existing diabetes

Oral hypoglycaemic agents are avoided in pregnancy. They cross the placenta and may provoke fetal hyperinsulinaemia.

The blood glucose levels return to normal within 48 hours of delivery (as cortisol and HPL levels fall). Those women with IGT who need insulin have an increased risk of developing diabetes (about 20% at 5 years, rising with each pregnancy), therefore follow-up is important (full GTT at 8 weeks).

The known diabetic

Before the introduction of insulin in 1922 maternal mortality for diabetics was 30% and 90% of babies died in utero.

Poorly controlled diabetes still causes many complications for mother and baby, and PNM can rise to 30% (ketoacidosis is rapidly lethal to the fetus); with perfect control (normal HbA_{1c} levels) the risks are little greater than for non-diabetics. Highest risk in those with microvascular complications prior to the pregnancy (e.g. retinopathy and nephropathy): these patients have an increased rate of complications in pregnancy (e.g. abruption, macrosomia, IUGR and hydramnios). With home glucose monitoring, admission to hospital is no longer necessary providing control is perfect and the pregnancy is normal. It is obviously essential that care is shared between the obstetrician and diabetic specialist in a joint clinic.

Preconception

The diabetic woman should be advised to start her family early, partly because of her decreased life expectancy and because PNM becomes very high if she develops complications (nephropathy, retinopathy). Her pregnancy should be planned and HbA_{1c} (glycosylated Hb) levels must be checked before stopping contraception (levels above 10% may significantly increase the chances of congenital abnormality).

Glycosylated Hb falls significantly in *normal* pregnancy from 9% to 3% due to increased RBC production. In well-controlled diabetes it will also fall in pregnancy.

Antenatal care

She should book early for antenatal care in a unit with an attached SCBU. An accurate assessment of gestation (early scan) is important for timing delivery and to implement good control of the diabetes. The motivation in these women is high and excellent diabetic control can be achieved with home monitoring using blood-testing strips (e.g. Dextrostix, BM Test, Visidex) together with a reflectance meter (e.g. Glucocheck, Glucometer, Hypocount). The aim is to keep preprandial plasma glucose below 6 mmol/l. In about a third of women the morning result is high (morning surge of cortisol and growth hormone) and yet increasing the teatime dose tends to cause nocturnal hypoglycaemia. This is solved by splitting the evening dose (Actrapid before tea; Insulatard at bedtime). May need × 3 or × 4 daily insulin regimens.

Educate family regarding treatment for 'hypos'. The baby is rarely at risk from hypo (unless accompanied by convulsions), therefore reassure on this point. Arrange fetal anomaly and growth scans. AFP should be unaffected by diabetes (may be slightly lower). Triple test (for Down's) is still of value in diabetics, but different reference ranges apply.

The woman should be seen in the clinic fortnightly to 32 weeks and then weekly to term. The insulin regimen should be changed to at least a b.d. regimen of a short-acting plus an intermediate-acting insulin, e.g. Actrapid and Insulatard. Human insulins may be advantageous (there is theoretical risk of antibodies to animal insulins which may cross the placenta and damage the fetal β-cells, possibly predisposing to diabetes in later life). Insulin requirements rise steadily from 12 to 32 weeks and fall sharply on delivery to pre-pregnancy doses (usually about half). Urine tests are unreliable in pregnancy. UTI more common so send MSUs regularly.

Fetal monitoring with 2- to 4-weekly scans is important because IUGR or macrosomia (big baby) can still occur even with good control, and can also occur in women who are not on insulin. Monitoring with CTG traces has so far failed to predict the intrauterine deaths that occur (not usually before 38 weeks) – fetal death has been described 12 hours after a normal CTG in diabetic and non-diabetic women. Biophysical profiles may be of use.

Labour

Best induced at 39 weeks because 2% of women have unexplained late intrauterine deaths. However, the incidence of RDS remains increased, particularly after caesarean delivery. Delivery is preferably by the vaginal route but the caesarean section rate is high for diabetics (30–50%) because the obstetrician tends to opt quickly for section if there are other complications (e.g. PET, malpresentation, long labour, twins, fetal distress).

During labour an i.v. infusion of 5% dextrose (11/12 hours) is given and i.v. infusion of insulin is started using a syringe pump. The insulin dose (usually 0.5–2 U/hour) is titrated against hourly blood glucose measurements (aiming for 4–5.5 mmol/l). 50 units of Actrapid in 50 ml of normal saline gives 1 U/h at 1 ml/hour. Patients rarely need more than 2–3 U/hour unless also having treatment for premature labour with i.v. sympathomimetics when doses of 16–20 U/hour may be needed. Hyperglycaemia must be avoided because glucose crosses the placenta, stimulating fetal islet cells and predisposing to neonatal hypoglycaemia.

Continuous CTG monitoring is performed in the usual way. A paediatrician should be present for the delivery.

Note: Steroids (to prevent RDS) should be used with the utmost caution in diabetics as significant hyperglycaemia will follow. The high incidence of RDS may benefit from very carefully supervised use in hospital with regular blood sugar assessment and recourse to i.v. regimens to keep the blood sugar from rising steeply, but not all authorities agree on this.

Post-delivery care

After delivery the i.v. insulin infusion dose should be halved and the infusion continued until the next main meal when the pre-pregnancy insulin dose can be given, or use a sliding scale.

The baby should be fed early (breast or bottle) and should remain with the mother. 8-hourly Dextrostix tests are performed for 48 hours to detect any neonatal hypoglycaemia.

The parents can be reassured that there is only a very small chance of the child ever developing diabetes (0.5%).

Contraception   The combined pill, POP or IUD are all suitable methods of contraception. Sterilisation is encouraged when appropriate. Only low-dose combined pills should be used, and because of the increased vascular risks they should only be used to delay conception for 2 years. Recurrent thrush may be a problem. There is some evidence that the IUD has higher infection and failure rates in diabetics.

With the advent of pre-pregnancy clinics, combined with diabetic/obstetric/neonatal developments, PNM in diabetics has fallen slowly. A major problem remains, however, with fetal anomalies and RDS.

◆ Thyroid disease

A goitre can occur in normal pregnancy because urinary iodide excretion tends to rise causing a relative lack of iodide and hyperplasia of the thyroid (the mechanism for which is uncertain). It can be prevented by the use of iodised salt in pregnancy.

Hypothyroidism   Hypothyroidism occurs in 1% of pregnancies, and has usually already been diagnosed because it tends to cause anovulatory infertility. In these patients the pre-pregnancy dose of thyroxine may need to be increased because of the increase in weight. However, mild hypothyroidism may present in pregnancy and may be suspected because of cold intolerance (unusual during pregnancy). It is diagnosed by a low FTI, low free thyroxine and raised TSH (specific TSH assay is best because HCG may cross-react and give falsely high TSH values) and it is treated with thyroxine (2 μg/kg body weight per day). Untreated hypothyroidism leads to a doubling in the stillbirth rate. Childhood hypothyroidism is not related to thyroid disease in the mother except in the case of rare enzyme defects.

Hyperthyroidism   Hyperthyroidism occurs in 1 in 500 pregnancies. Untreated, the fetal mortality rises to 50%. Mild hyperthyroidism does not reduce fertility. The diagnosis is suspected if there is poor weight gain or exophthalmos, especially with a family history of thyroid disease, and it is confirmed by a high free thyroxine and suppressed TSH. (**Note**: A small goitre, tachycardia, heat intolerance, palmar erythema, raised serum thyroxine and sometimes slightly elevated FTI can all occur in normal pregnancy.)

95% of cases are due to Graves disease which can be treated by subtotal thyroidectomy, or by carbimazole 15 mg t.d.s. reducing to once daily, to reduce the risk of fetal hypothyroidism. Carbimazole (and propylthiouracil) cross the placenta and can cause transient neonatal hypothyroidism and goitre. Long-term fetal effects are rare. Use the lowest dose that gives control. To reduce risk further, treatment can sometimes be stopped 3 weeks before delivery (carbimazole has a half-life of 3 days) although it must be restarted after delivery because there is a risk of a postnatal exacerbation of hyperthyroidism. The 'blocking-replacement regimen' (e.g. carbimazole + replacement thyroxine) should not be used in pregnancy. Breastfeeding is OK although small amounts do appear in the milk. Provided the baby is under surveillance this is not usually a problem.

Neonatal hyperthyroidism occurs in about 2% of the offspring due to high levels of thyroid stimulating antibodies crossing the placenta. It can be predicted by measuring anti-thyroid (stimulating) antibodies in the mother or suspected if there is a neonatal tachycardia in the last trimester. If the thyroid stimulating antibodies are known to be raised the maternal dose of carbimazole in pregnancy is kept high rather than as low as possible. (**Note**: Antibody levels can remain high with a past history of treated Graves disease.)

Neonatal thyrotoxicosis may not be apparent for several days. It causes restlessness, tachycardia, exophthalmos, goitre and feeding problems and is self-limiting, lasting about 2 months. It is treated with carbimazole and propranolol.

In summary, hyperthyroidism in pregnancy is best referred to a specialist clinic for monitoring and control by the lowest possible dose of anti-thyroid drugs. A past history still puts the baby at slight risk of neonatal thyrotoxicosis. Anti-thyroid drugs are not teratogenic.

Thyroid nodule   A solitary thyroid nodule in pregnancy can be diagnosed by USS/MRI scan (isotope scan is obviously contraindicated). If it is solid on ultrasound scan there is a 25% risk of malignancy. If the woman is euthyroid (i.e. it is not a toxic adenoma) needle biopsy or excision is indicated.

◆ Connective tissue disorders

Systemic lupus erythematosus (SLE)
Mainly affects women and its peak incidence is during the childbearing years. If it starts in pregnancy SLE can be easily confused with pre-eclampsia, and in severe cases of PET it should be excluded by measuring DNA-binding antibody levels. SLE causes renal damage with proteinuria and sometimes hypertension but, unlike PET, causes skin rashes, joint and pleuritic symptoms and tends to worsen rather than remit after delivery. SLE is strongly associated with recurrent abortions, IUGR/intrauterine death, and premature labour and PNM are increased. Self-limiting neonatal SLE can occur rarely, due to antibodies crossing the placenta (rashes, haemolysis, fetal or neonatal complete heart-block). Patients with active SLE should defer pregnancy until in remission.

Steroid therapy throughout pregnancy is usually safe (cleft palate, NTD, growth retardation and neonatal adrenal insufficiency are slightly increased). Steroid administration should be increased during delivery and for relapses, e.g. hydrocortisone 100 mg i.v. every 8 hours. Azathioprine is also useful, particularly when arteritis is a feature. Low-dose aspirin, 75 mg daily, is of value when started early (at first positive pregnancy test). Thromboprophylaxis is sometimes indicated as the risk of venous and arterial thrombosis is increased in all these conditions.

Other related autoimmune disorders
Ask at booking about any history of rheumatic or skin-joint problems as well as previous renal disease. Pregnancy is often the first time a women has ever had her urine tested, blood pressure taken or FBC checked.

Test mother for antinuclear, anticardiolipin, and antiphospholipid antibodies. *Antiphospholipid syndrome (APLS)* is increasingly recognised as a cause of poor pregnancy outcome. Management is as for SLE. A rare condition, *ANCA vasculitis,* presents with renal and skin involvement (look specifically for anti-DNA and ANCA antibodies).

◆ Other medical conditions in pregnancy

Focal migraine/
hemiplegic migraine

Focal migraine with alarming prodromal symptoms of hemiplegia or hemisensory change can present for the first time in pregnancy. After a few hours the onset of severe headache and nausea usually makes the diagnosis obvious. It is a benign condition in pregnancy not associated with subsequent arterial occlusion. Differential diagnosis is vital by an expert to exclude intracranial thrombosis: CT scan if in doubt.

Glomerulonephritis

Up to 50% of women presenting with hypertension or proteinuria in pregnancy have been shown to have underlying renal disease in studies where renal biopsies have been performed. It is important to exclude this possibility because the condition can deteriorate sharply in pregnancy and occasionally precipitates renal failure. Urine microscopy provides the best test for glomerulonephritis: increased counts of glomerular erythrocytes of bizarre shape and size is a sensitive and specific indicator of glomerulonephritis. Renal biopsy is usually deferred until after pregnancy. Serial serum albumin and creatinine, creatinine clearance and 24-hour urinary protein excretion measurements are useful in monitoring progress. BP may be labile in acute renal disease and should be watched closely.

Toxic erythema

The most common rash of pregnancy (1 in 20). Red, itchy, oedematous papules and plaques, starting on abdominal striae and spreading to the arms and legs. Usually occurs in late third trimester and tends to recur in subsequent pregnancies. Skin immunofluorescence is negative. It can resemble erythema multiforme. Check liver function and platelet count – increased AST is associated with IUGR and pre-eclampsia.

Herpes gestationis

Rare (about 1 in 5000 pregnancies). Resembles urticarial papules and plaques but, in addition, tense thick-walled blisters occur, which may be haemorrhagic. Appears at any time in pregnancy or puerperium and usually subsides within a month of delivery. Immunofluorescence shows complement deposition along the basement membrane. The infant may be born with a similar rash. Severe eruptions are treated with steroids. It tends to recur in subsequent pregnancies.

Acute fatty liver of
pregnancy

This condition is very rare (1 in 10 000). The patient usually presents in late pregnancy with abdominal pain, vomiting and then jaundice. DIC and renal failure occur. *Maternal mortality is 80%* and PNM 70%. The patient deteriorates quickly and can die within 1–2 days of presentation. Management is by immediate delivery and hepatic support with transfusion of blood and fresh frozen plasma, and maintenance of the blood sugar (hypoglycaemia is common and exacerbates the condition). Acute fatty liver is characterised by a polymorph leucocytosis, often with only mildly elevated liver function tests, together

with mild hypertension and proteinuria. Liver biopsy shows fatty droplets (PET shows petechiae and fibrinoid necrosis). The *differential diagnosis* includes:
– cholestasis of pregnancy
– biliary obstruction
– acute viral or drug-induced hepatitis
– severe PET with greatly raised transaminases
– haemolytic uraemic syndrome
– thrombotic thrombocytopenic purpura

Autoimmune thrombocytopenic purpura (ITP)

This is less common than benign gestational thrombocytopenia. A platelet count of $120–150 \times 10^9/l$ is fairly common in the third trimester. Counts below this or which have fallen suddenly should be investigated.

ITP has a significant incidence of maternal, fetal (10%) and neonatal (5%) deaths. Known cases may have had a splenectomy (and be on prophylactic penicillin) before getting pregnant. Maternal haemorrhage is unlikely if the platelet count is $>50 \times 10^9/l$ at delivery. Transplacental IgG causes neonatal thrombocytopenia in 50% of cases, which is worst 2–5 days after birth when the fetal splenic circulation becomes established.

Bleeding at delivery is likely to occur if the platelet count is persistently below $20 \times 10^9/l$, although the fetal risk at this level is still only 10–15%. Levels above this in asymptomatic women may be observed and pregnancy should be allowed to continue. High-dose steroids and platelet infusions often fail to raise the platelet count in pregnancy. Immunoglobulin infusions may improve platelet function, but the benefits are unproven and their use has become uncommon. Measure anti-platelet antibodies to monitor progress (and assess the fetal risk). The fetal platelet count can be measured by FBS in labour if anticipating vaginal delivery, but the level at which vaginal delivery should be avoided (because of the risk of intracranial haemorrhage in the baby) is uncertain.

Addison's disease

In treated Addison's disease fertility is normal. The patient should already know to increase cortisol (but not fludrocortisone) intake at times of stress or fever. If vomiting occurs the patient needs 100 mg i.m. hydrocortisone as well as an anti-emetic, e.g. prochlorperazine (Stemetil) as a 25 mg suppository or 12.5 mg intramuscularly. Arrange urgent admission if vomiting does not settle. During labour she will need 100 mg hydrocortisone i.m. every 6 hours. She can be reassured that replacement doses of hydrocortisone and fludrocortisone are not teratogenic.

Major haemoglobinopathies

Sickle cell disease (Hb SS) and sickle cell thalassaemia (Hb SC)

Hb SS: homozygous sickle cell *disease* in pregnancy is rare as many die young or are infertile. There is increased maternal and perinatal

mortality and morbidity due to:
- miscarriage
- IUGR
- preterm labour
- severe pre-eclampsia
- thromboembolic complications

Placental infarction leads to abortion (18%), stillbirth (12%) and IUGR. Pre-eclampsia and urinary infections are common, but maternal *mortality* is now negligible. Current management involves prophylactic iron (stores are often low despite classic teaching on haemolysis), folic acid 5 mg daily throughout pregnancy, prompt treatment of infections, and exchange transfusions from 28 weeks to reduce the level of haemoglobin S below 40%. Simple transfusions, with diuretics, can be used if the patient is already anaemic (Hb < 7 g/dl) due to splenic sequestration. Painful sickling crises (pulmonary and bone infarcts) tend to occur in late pregnancy and are treated with opiate analgesics, O_2 and rehydration. Delivery should be vaginal. Tubal ligation should be advised on completing the family. Temporary contraception should be reliable (e.g. IUD, despite risk of infection).

Hb SC is more common than Hb SS and usually milder but massive sickling crises still occur, especially in the puerperium. May be diagnosed for the first time in pregnancy. There are usually few complications in pregnancy but it is associated with more thrombosis. Check haemoglobin electrophoresis of both parents: prenatal screening and diagnosis is possible. Consider low-dose heparin prophylaxis for operative delivery (as thromboembolic complications are more common). If chest pain develops in late pregnancy or the puerperium pulmonary embolus should be assumed and urgent exchange transfusion is indicated.

Sickle cell trait (Hb AS) Occurs in 10% of Caribbean populations and 20% of West Africans. It has no effect on maternal or perinatal mortality. There is an increased incidence of urinary infections and haematuria (sickling in renal medulla). It is important to warn the anaesthetist as tissue infarcts can occur with poor hydration or inadequate oxygen levels. Prenatal screening of the partner is important.

Note: Sickling tests must be carried out on all women of appropriate racial background, and if positive the partner must be checked. Prenatal diagnosis should be considered if both partners carry traits. The infant's blood must be tested by electrophoresis immediately after birth.

Thalassaemia Thalassaemias are characterised by abnormal globin chain synthesis in the haemoglobin molecule. Thalassaemias are classified as α or β depending on which globin chain is affected. The major obstetric issue is prenatal screening and diagnosis. All are recessively inherited. Different mutations are specific to certain populations, hence ethnic differences in prevalance.

α *thalassaemias.* Commonest in SE Asia.
- heterozygous (trait): are asymptomatic but anaemic in pregnancy
- homozygous: variable effects from intrauterine death with hydrops (this is, interestingly, a rare cause of severe early-onset

pre eclampsia in the mother), to variable haemolytic anaemia in adult life. Most serious α-thalassaemias are fatal

β-thalassaemias: Common in the Eastern Mediterranean, Middle East, India and SE Asia.
- minor (trait): common. Leads to anaemia in pregnancy. Must avoid iron overload so no parenteral iron, but oral Fe + folate is safe. In severe cases transfuse
- major: these women rarely achieve pregnancy as survival to adulthood requires repeated transfusions to avoid bony deformities due to poor bone growth (because of relative hypoxia), and these lead to liver, myocardial and endocrine organ damage from iron overload

Screening for thalassaemias: do Hb, MCV and electrophoresis in appropriate ethnic groups, unless across-the-board screening is funded locally.

Malaria   Malaria in pregnancy is more severe than usual, with risks of abortion and premature labour (and rarely of transplacental transmission). Acute malaria in a pregnant woman requires speedy and complete treatment by the most effective drugs available, which are much less hazardous to mother and fetus than severe malaria.

Chemoprophylaxis is essential for a pregnant woman visiting an endemic area. Increasing resistance to the drugs together with possible side-effects on the fetus mean that up-to-date advice must be sought on the best drug for a particular area (check with the Institute for Tropical Medicine, London). Chloroquine is the least harmful and usually the best choice, and will give fair protection in resistant areas. The dose of chloroquine is 300 mg once weekly (including 1 week before and 6 weeks after travelling). Congenital abnormalities do not occur at this dosage. Babies need the usual protection from mosquito bites (nets, space sprays) because chloroquine appears only in small quantities in breast milk.

◆ Iron-deficiency anaemia

The importance of severe anaemia is that PNM is doubled and PPH becomes life-threatening.

Anaemia in pregnancy is defined as an Hb below 10 g/dl. The red cell mass is increased by 20% in pregnancy but the plasma volume rises by about 30%: the Hb concentration therefore falls due to relative haemodilution and the fall is more marked as pregnancy advances:
1st trimester – 12.5 g/dl
2nd trimester – 11.5 g/dl
term   – 11.0 g/dl

There is a wide variation in plasma volume changes. A low–normal Hb (10–11 g/dl) with a normal MCV and MCH suggests the cause is simply haemodilution – check ferritin to assess iron stores.

Demand for iron in pregnancy:
    fetus and placenta   – 400 mg
    increased maternal RBCs – 200 mg

haemorrhage – 200 mg
lactation   – 200 mg

100 mg (9 × 11 mg) is saved by absent menstruation and iron absorption is increased in pregnancy. Iron-deficiency anaemia is becoming less common but occurs if the woman has had *heavy periods or frequently recurring pregnancies*. It is common in the tropics due to poor diet and hookworms (where malaria and sickle cell anaemia may lower the Hb further).

The iron stores of the liver and spleen amount to about 1000 mg. Without prophylaxis iron stores in the bone marrow, however, will be largely exhausted by term and Fe prophylaxis in mid-pregnancy is advocated by most obstetricians. Prophylaxis from 12–36 weeks will maintain iron stores, e.g. Pregaday (100 mg elemental iron as ferrous fumarate and 350 μg of folate). Iron-deficiency anaemia is diagnosed by a low Hb with:
– low MCV (<76), low MCH (<28)
– hypochromic microcytic film
– low serum iron with a raised TIBC (diagnostic)
– low serum ferritin (reflecting low stores)

Management

Any severe anaemia, even in early pregnancy, needs full investigation prior to treatment.

Mild anaemia (Hb 9–10 g/dl) is initially assumed to be due to iron deficiency and treated with 'double iron', i.e. twice the prophylactic dosage. Hb should rise at the rate of 0.5 g/dl per week. Iron should be continued for 3 months postpartum. If there is no response (reticulocytes should rise after 10 days), serum iron, TIBC and ferritin are measured and other causes must be excluded:
– chronic UTI (depressed erythropoietin, high ferritin)
– thalassaemia minor (very low MCV, Hb electrophoresis)
– megaloblastic anaemia (serum B_{12} and folate) – rare in UK unless coeliac
– continued bleeding (stools for occult blood and parasites)

Mild anaemia resistant to iron:
– check no haemoglobinopathy, e.g. thalassaemia trait
– check compliance (serum ferritin)

Parenteral iron does not increase the rate of *synthesis* of haemoglobin and is only indicated if iron-deficiency anaemia (Hb <9 g/dl) is still present at 32 weeks, due to malabsorption (no rise in serum iron measured after an oral iron load), to true intolerance or to lack of compliance of oral iron. Jectofer (iron sorbitol) is given by deep i.m. injection – usually 100 mg (2 ml) a day for about 7 days. It is painful and can cause headache, nausea and a metallic taste in the mouth for several hours afterwards. It should not be given if the patient has a UTI (it increases pyuria).

Intravenous infusion using iron sucrose (Venofer) is less painful but can be life-threatening if anaphylaxis. Oral iron must be stopped for 2 days beforehand. *Anaphylaxis* occurs rarely but may prove fatal, and a test dose must be given first (with i.v. adrenaline, Piriton, hydrocortisone and facilities for intubation and resuscitation to hand).

Transfusion is needed occasionally for severe anaemia after 36 weeks, especially if heavy blood loss is likely at delivery (e.g. placenta praevia). All patients should have an Hb of at least 10 g/dl at the onset of labour. 1 unit of packed cells gives a rise in Hb of 1 g/dl. Transfusion should be accompanied by correction of the dietary deficiency.

◆ Urinary tract infection

Urinary tract infection is more common in pregnancy because of stasis in the dilated and partially obstructed ureters (progesterone and pelvic mass), increased vesico-ureteric reflux, and stasis in the upper ureter (especially the right) due to pressure from the uterus in late pregnancy.

About 6% of pregnant women have *asymptomatic bacteriuria* ($>10^5$ organisms per ml). This can be screened for routinely with a booking MSU and treated with appropriate antibiotics. Recheck after 1 week off antibiotics – it recurs in 35%:
- they have about a 30% chance of developing acute pyelonephritis
- if it is recurrent, there is a strong possibility that they have an underlying chronic pyelonephritis or renal tract abnormality (also said to be more likely if antibiotics fail to cure associated pyuria) and renal ultrasound is indicated. Consider repeat USS 3 months after delivery, once the ureters are a normal size again
- it probably increases the chance of premature labour

Note: In 1955 Kass showed that an MSU (after thorough skin cleaning) with 10^5 organisms per ml had an 80% chance of detecting bladder infection, and two positive MSUs a 96% chance. A catheter specimen of urine has a 99% chance of being correct. A single high dose of a broad-spectrum antibiotic is often just as effective as a 5-day course and is less likely to cause thrush.

Asymptomatic bacteriuria *in non-pregnant women* seems to be common and transient and probably needs no treatment.

Acute pyelonephritis: 50% have had preceding asymptomatic bacteriuria. It may present merely with nausea and malaise or with high fever, rigors, renal tenderness and dysuria. The dangers are fetal demise or premature labour and permanent maternal renal damage. Take an MSU and treat promptly with i.v. ampicillin, i.v. fluids, aspirin and temperature control measures. Anaemia commonly occurs afterwards (decreased erythropoietin). Follow-up MSUs are needed throughout pregnancy, e.g. monthly.

Two proven UTIs is an indication to begin continuous low-dose prophylaxis, e.g. ampicillin, trimethoprim or nitrofurantoin. Co-trimoxazole is contraindicated in late pregnancy because of the sulphonamide component, which causes neonatal hyperbilirubinaemia.

◆ Heart disease

Affects about 1% of pregnant women, corrected congenital heart disease now being much more common than rheumatic. A *murmur* may be first detected at routine examination on booking: most are innocent flow murmurs from the hyperdynamic circulation.

Mitral stenosis causes a small-volume pulse, loud first sound, opening snap (which resembles a loud split second sound) and a soft rumbling mid-diastolic murmur localised to the apex.

Most congenital heart disease causes an obvious systolic murmur (VSD, aortic stenosis, coarctation, patent ductus). Atrial septal defect causes a fixed split second sound and a pulmonary flow murmur and eventually causes pulmonary hypertension.

Note: A soft ejection murmur, oedema, slight dyspnoea and left axis deviation are normal in pregnancy. Cardiac output increases significantly by 12 weeks gestation. If no maternal compromise by this time, prognosis is good. The next most worrying time is the third stage of labour as sudden increase in pre-load may cause failure.

Heart disease in pregnancy is not usually an indication for termination or elective section. Combined care with a cardiologist is necessary. With good management there should be no deterioration in the heart condition. PNM is only increased with cyanotic congenital heart disease. Delivery may involve transfer to a unit with cardiac anaesthesia facilities for the mother in case of intrapartum complications, or for the immediate care of a newborn expected to have congenital heart disease.

Severe heart disease accounts for <10% of maternal mortality. Significant maternal mortality is particularly associated with Marfan's syndrome, inoperable cyanotic congenital heart disease, primary pulmonary hypertension and congestive cardiomyopathy. Any of these conditions may be a medical indication for termination of pregnancy.

Pregnancy increases the blood volume by 30% and cardiac output (stroke volume × rate) by 30% from 12 weeks to term. Increased flow across a narrow valve increases the chance of *LVF* developing and increased rest is important – strict bed-rest throughout pregnancy is necessary if LVF develops. The risk of LVF is highest just after delivery of the placenta as 500 ml of blood is squeezed out of the uterus into the circulation. Ergometrine (which increases diastolic BP by 10–15 mmHg) should be avoided.

Assessing the degree of *dyspnoea on exertion* is a poor guide to cardiac behaviour in pregnancy and does not help to predict the main complications which are LVF and SBE. Increasing dyspnoea can be difficult to interpret (anaemia, hypertension, arrythmias and chest infection) and is normal in advanced pregnancy: the patient needs detailed assessment including echocardiography and oxygen saturation measurements.

Mitral valvotomy is very rarely necessary in pregnancy but can be performed at any stage – preferably after 12 weeks to decrease the chance of miscarriage.

In patients with *prosthetic heart valves* the risk of thromboembolism is increased. If warfarin therapy is well controlled the risks to the woman are low but there is a risk of teratogenesis (worst at 6–9 weeks) and of fetal intracranial haemorrhage and an increased risk of spontaneous abortion. The patient should be admitted at least 2 weeks before delivery in order to stop warfarin and start i.v. heparin before labour (heparin does not cross the placenta). Heparin is then reversed for the delivery and restarted immediately afterwards. If labour starts unexpectedly on warfarin the woman is given fresh frozen plasma and the baby vitamin K. The risk of an abnormal baby (CNS micro-haemorrhages) is less than 10%.

Management
- avoid smoking
- treat infections and give antibiotic prophylaxis for procedures (e.g. amnio, cervical suture, instrumental delivery)
- treat anaemia and infections vigorously. If fever occurs, consider endocarditis and take blood cultures
- daily rest, see fortnightly, see cardiologist at 28 weeks (re-echo)
- digoxin, diuretics, anti-arrhythmics and warfarin/heparin are used as necessary. Plasma digoxin levels should be measured in those who fail to respond. Warfarin (fibrillation or valve prosthesis) is stopped at 37 weeks and heparin infusion started (warfarin crosses the placenta and increases the chance of intracranial haemorrhage in the fetus)
- labour can be induced as normal for obstetric indications
- prophylactic antibiotics to cover delivery (e.g. amoxicillin 1 g i.v. in labour and 500 mg orally 6 hours later + gentamicin 120 mg i.v. after delivery)
- adequate pain relief is important. Any tachycardia (anaemia, infection, fibrillation, pain, fear) increases the chance of LVF developing. Epidural should be avoided if BP is already low. May cause increased pre-load by giving fluids
- short second stage with elective forceps. Avoid ergometrine if there is a risk of LVF (Syntocinon 5 units i.v. is preferred)
- thromboprophylaxis
- adequate hydration and encourage early ambulation
- discuss contraception. If LVF developed in pregnancy, sterilisation is advised

◆ Infections and the fetus

The most important infections in pregnancy are:
- CMV
- toxoplasmosis
- chickenpox
- herpes
- hepatitis B
- parvovirus
- rubella
- HIV
- syphilis

Note: It is important to remember that many sequelae of *viral infection* are *not* detectable by screening tests such as USS (e.g. deafness, blindness, mental retardation). Fetal sampling by cordocentesis will confirm viraemia in the fetus but *not* predict the severity of any sequelae. Counselling and advice can therefore be extremely difficult. Seek expert advice.

Common viral infections

The fetus is infected via the mother and *most fetal infections are viral* (except syphilis and toxoplasmosis). Cellular immunity is decreased in pregnancy and the effect of viral infections on the mother can be more severe than usual, especially polio. Nevertheless, there is no evidence that *influenza, mumps* or *measles* specifically damage the fetus although reports of the latter in pregnancy are rare. High fever of any cause, however, increases the risk of abortion or stillbirth.

Primary CMV infection

Can damage the fetus. The mother is usually asymptomatic (rarely it mimics glandular fever) and the only way to demonstrate an infection would be serial serology to observe seroconversion. No vaccine is available and nothing can be done to prevent infection, although known seronegative pregnant women should not nurse infants with overt CMV disease because the infant can excrete the virus for several months. Congenital infection occurs in 1% of live births and damages about 1 in 1000. The effects on the fetus can be:
– apparently none (the majority)
– malformations (microcephaly, retardation, deafness, fits, choroiditis)
– stillbirth
– active infection (jaundice, hepatosplenomegaly, purpura)
– low birth weight

In some centres women are screened for CMV antibodies and seronegative women are asked to report any fevers, so serology can be checked.

Toxoplasmosis

One-third of women in the UK of reproductive age are seropositive (for IgG, signifying previous infection). Numbers are greater in France and Northern Europe where screening programmes are different. About 0.2% of women acquire the disease during pregnancy and in about 10% of these the fetus is damaged. The infection is acquired from cat faeces or from raw meat. The mother may only have a transient fever. The best method of diagnosing acute infection is by assay of the specific IgM by an enzyme-linked immunosorbent assay. The effects on the fetus may be:
– apparently none (except positive serology)
– stillbirth
– malformation (microcephaly, retardation, fits)
– active infection (jaundice, hepatomegaly, purpura)

No live vaccine is available.

Fortunately, one attack gives immunity and subsequent children are normal. Screening is possible in early pregnancy and again in 20 weeks, if negative. Women undergoing seroconversion can be offered spiramycin which is thought to reduce risk.

Chickenpox

Infection with the varicella-zoster virus is rare (5/100 000 pregnancies) in pregnancy because most women (>95%) have had it in childhood but when it occurs it tends to be severe. *Varicella pneumonitis* is the major maternal complication, causes maternal mortality of up to 40% (contrast with 15% mortality without aciclovir in the non-pregnant) and requires intensive medical intervention and support. *Varicella embryopathy* is rare, causing mainly skin, eye and

CNS lesions. There are no good studies confirming transplacental passage of varicella virus. Varicella can, however, cause breaks in the chromosomal material which may predispose to later development of malignancies in affected fetuses, especially leukaemias, although these cases are rare. Non-immune pregnant women in contact with or who develop varicella-zoster should receive VZIG and aciclovir as soon as possible, although it remains difficult to prove fetal benefit.

The risks to the fetus of maternal chickenpox infection in the few days/weeks before delivery are much greater than the chance of teratogenesis when the infection is contracted in the first trimester. *Neonatal varicella has a 30% mortality rate.* Maternal IgG crosses the placenta and this passage is protective. Neonatal risk therefore depends on the timing of the infection relative to the delivery.

Note: The mother is viraemic 10–17 days *after* exposure to the virus and 12–48 hours *before* development of the rash. VZ antibodies appear 4–5 days after the rash develops. Maternal VZIG will also be of some benefit to the newborn if >5 days elapsed *before* delivery – delivery, if elective, should be delayed. *All infants born to women developing varicella within one week of delivery should receive VZIG at birth.*

Genital herpes

A primary attack of genital herpes in pregnancy can rarely cause fetal malformations (microcephaly, choroiditis) or active disease (encephalitis, hepatitis) and primary herpes in late pregnancy can be an indication for delivery by section, unless membranes have already been ruptured for many hours (in which case there is no proven benefit in reducing encephalitis). Better to look for active lesions on the cervix on admission in labour or go by history alone, although weekly viral swabs from 32 weeks may be helpful in reassuring the patient about vaginal delivery.

Hepatitis

There is no evidence that hepatitis A or B causes congenital abnormalities. Infection in pregnancy is not an indication for termination, but transplacental and intrapartum infection occurs. Maternal screening looks for HB_sAg (surface antigen), but infectivity is determined by the presence of e antigen (HB_eAg). Highest risk to carers and the fetus is when the mother is e antigen positive but e antibody negative. Check maternal HB surface *and* e antigen/antibody status in high-risk groups (e.g. intravenous drug abusers, Vietnamese refugees).

If the mother develops clinical hepatitis B in late pregnancy or the puerperium, the infant is in danger of catching the infection from contact with maternal blood at delivery and should be given specific HB_sAg immunoglobulin after birth.

Asymptomatic carriers of hepatitis B can infect their baby transplacentally or at delivery, especially if they are e antigen positive and antibody negative. Breastfeeding is not contraindicated. The babies must be given 200 μg IgG i.m. as soon as possible after delivery – always within 48 hrs, plus HB vaccine 10 μg in the opposite arm at the same time. Babies are followed up at 1 and 6 months for further doses of HB vaccine, and at 1 year for LFTs and HB_sAg titre. Women who are e antigen positive should remain under lifelong follow-up by a physician with an interest in liver disease.

Parvovirus infection

Common in the wider community (slap-face rash in school-age children).

The infection is usually asymptomatic in mothers, but can cause malaise, rash, and fever.

Risks to the fetus are worst if contracted before 24 weeks, especially with the *B19 type* virus. Causes temporary aplastic crisis in fetus leading to severe anaemia and hydrops (ascites, oedema, cardiac failure – USS). If recognised, intrauterine transfusions (as for Rhesus) can maintain fetal haemoglobin while the marrow recovers. There have been no recorded cases of mental or physical long-term handicap in a few treated cases. Need to scan weekly for 8–10 weeks after contact to check for hydrops. Parvovirus after 26 weeks seems to cause fewer problems. Parvovirus is probably underestimated as a cause of non-immune hydrops.

Rubella

In 1941 Gregg, an Australian ophthalmologist, noticed 68 cases of congenital cataract following an epidemic of rubella, and other congenital abnormalities were soon recognised. In 1962 the virus was isolated and in 1969 the live attenuated vaccine was introduced.

Rubella antibodies are screened at booking. MMR vaccination for all children (boys *and* girls) at 13 months and at pre-school age, with specific rubella vaccination of girls who have been missed at age 11–14 is the practice in the UK, but some girls are still missed. Ideally, all women should have preconception rubella screening (e.g. when prescribing the pill). A history of 'German measles' is an unreliable guide to immune status.

If a woman of unknown immunity is in contact with rubella during the first trimester of pregnancy, take blood immediately for antibodies (IgG measured by single radial haemolysis) and repeat in 10 days (see Table 5).

If a woman already has antibodies she is immune. However, if it is more than 2 weeks since the contact or if she has had a recent rubella-like illness, then the specific test (for IgM) should also be performed because a raised IgG may be due to present rather than past infection. Take throat swabs and stools for virology (within 2 days of fever or rash). If positive, consider abortion, depending on gestation.

The *chances of congenital damage* are:
– 50% at 4 weeks
– 25% at 8 weeks
– 15% at 12 weeks (deafness only)

The fetus may be stillborn or born with active infection (often IUGR + purpura, hepatosplenomegaly, jaundice, encephalitis) or have

Table 6 Testing for rubella antibodies in pregnancy

1st test	2nd test	Action
+	Unnecessary	None
–	–	Immunise in puerperium
–	+	Counselling *re* anomalies. ?TOP

congenital abnormalities:
– cataract
– patient ductus (or ASD or PS)
– high-tone deafness
– microcephaly, cerebral palsy
– microphthalmia

If the woman has no antibodies she is immunised in the puerperium with live attenuated rubella vaccine.

Breastfeeding is allowed following vaccination but pregnancy should be avoided for 3 months – medroxyprogesterone 150 mg i.m. can be given simultaneously (although there have been no adverse reports, of women getting pregnant recently after vaccination and this is not usually a reason for TOP). A mild reaction (fever, rash, lymphadenopathy, arthralgia) sometimes occurs about 9 days after vaccination.

Contraindications to the live vaccine are:
– known pregnancy
– immunosuppression
– fever or infection
– thrombocytopenia (drop in platelet count following vaccination has been reported)
– allergy to neomycin, polymixin (in the vaccine)

Note: Specific gammaglobulin during pregnancy does *not* help to protect the infant and is not used even if a seronegative pregnant woman has contact with rubella.

The risk of malformation after inadvertant vaccination in pregnancy is very low and it is not an indication for termination.

HIV   HIV can be transmitted from mother to child transplacentally, at delivery or via breast milk. Without antiviral therapy the risk of transmission is around 20% in the UK (even if breastfeeding is avoided) – mostly during the third trimester and at delivery. Routine antenatal screening has been widespread in the UK from mid-2000: specific Government funding has been allocated. In most UK regions the prevalence of HIV is low (higher in inner cities).

With appropriate antenatal and intrapartum care, transmission is reduced to <5%. Monitor maternal CD4 count and total viral load. If CD4 count is <200/mm^3, zidovudine monotherapy given orally in the second and third trimesters, and i.v. for delivery, plus treatment of the baby until 6 weeks of age, reduces transmission by two-thirds. If the woman is receiving triple therapy for more advanced disease continue in pregnancy (drug safety data more limited, however).

Caesarean delivery with intact membranes is advised – transmission to the infant can occur through ingestion of maternal secretions and blood at vaginal delivery.

Breastfeeding should be avoided – increases transmission by approx 15% in HIV carriers.

Syphilis   Primary syphilis occurs rarely in the UK, but may present as a vulval ulcer. *Treponema pallidum* readily crosses the placenta to infect the fetus. At birth hepatosplenomegaly and jaundice may be present. Bony changes are present in >90% affected newborns. Do MHA-TP (microhaemagglutination assay for *T. pallidum* antibodies) if high VDRL titre. False-positive VDRL results occur with yaws. Congenital syphilis can be prevented by treatment with benzylpenicillin throughout the pregnancy.

◆ Rhesus disease

15% of women in the UK are Rhesus-negative (dd): if the father is homozygous Rhesus-positive (DD) the baby will be Rhesus-positive; if he is heterozygous (Dd) there is a 50% chance that the baby will be Rhesus-positive. Fetal red cells cross into the maternal circulation during delivery, therapeutic and spontaneous abortion, ectopics, APH, amniocentesis, severe abdominal trauma (including seat belt injury: shearing forces between placenta and uterine wall), external version or caesarean section and will stimulate maternal antibody production. (Rhesus-positive transfusions will also produce antibodies.)

Clinical assessment

Rhesus-negative women without antibodies: blood is taken at booking, at 28 and at 34 weeks to screen for antibodies. At delivery, cord blood is taken for blood group and Coombs' test (to confirm that the cells are not coated with antibodies) and maternal blood is taken (to estimate the number of fetal cells in it by the acid elution of maternal haemoglobin – the Kleihauer test).

Rhesus-negative women with antibodies: these pregnancies are becoming rare and are best managed in special centres. The antibodies are IgG and cross back to the fetus causing haemolysis which can lead to:
- anaemia
- high-output cardiac failure
- oedema and ascites (hydrops)
- hepatosplenomegaly (increased fetal haemopoiesis)
- early neonatal jaundice
- kernicterus (should never occur with good SCBU management)

Fortnightly maternal blood antibody estimations are performed from the time they are first detected and the partner's genotype confirmed. The severity of the effect on the fetus is difficult to predict from maternal antibody levels alone. If levels are high (>4–10 IU) or rapidly rising, then fetal blood sampling by serial cordocentesis is indicated to determine the fetal Hb, haematocrit, genotype, antibody level and bilirubin level. (Historically, amniotic fluid was used and the bilirubin level plotted against gestation on a Liley chart to judge the severity of the disease.)

The severity of the disease is *judged by serial measurements*:
- serum anti-D levels (poor guide)
- scans (accumulation of ascites/hydrops)
- fetal blood sampling

Management

Involves referral to a specialist centre for:
- fetal scans (growth and ascites)
- intrauterine transfusions of Rhesus-negative blood, preferably directly into the umbilical cord (intra-abdominal fetal transfusion

141

can be easier at late gestations, but is technically difficult before 23 weeks and the fetal mortality is higher)
– antenatal steroids and delivery at 34 weeks (or sooner): crossmatch blood for the baby based on mother's sample
– maternal plasmapheresis (very rarely used)

In a few women with high anti-D levels fetal hydrops develops before 23 weeks. In these cases direct umbilical cord sampling and transfusion can be undertaken as early as 18 weeks by *cordocentesis*.

With the reduced mortality in neonatal intensive care units there is a tendency to deliver early, even at 29–30 weeks, rather than risk intrauterine transfusion.

At delivery, cord blood is taken for haemoglobin, grouping, bilirubin and Coombs' test (to confirm the diagnosis). Bilirubin can no longer be removed by the placenta and starts to rise immediately after delivery causing *jaundice* and the possibility of kernicterus. The baby will begin phototherapy immediately.

Bilirubin is monitored on SCBU and *exchange transfusion* is necessary if it rises rapidly. 'Top-up' transfusions may be needed later for anaemia. Also give iron and vitamins in early infant months.

Prevention of Rhesus immunisation

500 IU of anti-D is usually given within 72 hours of delivery (250 IU is usually sufficient if gestation was up to 20 weeks, e.g. after miscarriage, amnio, etc.), but a higher dose may be needed if large numbers of fetal cells are found in maternal blood. Always do a Kleihauer test when giving anti-D for events after 20 weeks and await lab advice in case additional doses are required.

New RCOG guidelines (1999) state that anti-D may be omitted for potentially sensitising events at gestations below 12 weeks, unless surgical evacuation of the uterus has occurred. Many units, however, continue to use anti-D at all gestations. The anti-D coats and destroys the fetal cells and prevents sensitisation of the mother's immune system.

Giving anti-D routinely to all Rh-negative women immediately after delivery has largely been replaced by prompt checking of the baby's group and giving it only if the baby is Rh-positive: the results reporting and follow-up mechanism must be absolutely foolproof and enable anti-D to be given within 72 hours maximum. Most anti-D now comes from US donors or using new biotechnology methods, reducing earlier anxieties about BSE and UK donors.

Unrecognised sensitising events can cause significant immunisation of a Rh-negative woman and so Rhesus incompatibility complications will continue to be seen. The RCOG guidelines therefore advise routine prophylaxis to *all* Rh-negative women at 28 and 34 weeks but many health authorities will not yet fund this. The number of cases saved would be small, but each is hugely costly.

Anti-D is *not* indicated if:
– the baby is known to be Rh-negative
– the mother already has antibodies or has received anti-D within 6 weeks and the Kleihauer test is negative

The current prophylaxis programme still fails to prevent about 500 Rh-negative women becoming immunised each year, because of:
- failure to give anti-D
- failure of anti-D to be effective
- intrapartum immunisation

There can be no excuse for forgetting to give anti-D after abortion (therapeutic or spontaneous). Failure of anti-D to prevent maternal immunisation occurs either because insufficient anti-D is given or because intrapartum sensitisation has occurred before postpartum anti-D is indicated. The Kleihauer test (fetal cell count) estimates the size of any transplacental haemorrhage and this is particularly important after complications such as abruption, manual removal of the placenta and fulminant eclampsia.

Note: 500 IU anti-D 'neutralises' 4 ml fetal red cells.

◆ Antepartum haemorrhage (APH)

Defined as vaginal bleeding after 28 weeks (but if the fetus may be viable, i.e. from 24 weeks, management is the same). THE CARDINAL RULE is to admit the woman and *never perform a vaginal examination until ultrasound scan has excluded placenta praevia.*

The *possible causes* are:
- placenta praevia
- placental abruption
- incidental (cervix: ectropion, polyp or tumour)
- rare causes – vasa praevia, trauma

Placenta praevia

Classically presents as recurrent painless bleeds, especially around 30–32 weeks as the lower segment forms. It may be unprovoked or follow intercourse. Typically the head is high, may deviate to one side and does not descend onto the pelvic brim when the woman stands up. Transverse or breech presentation may occur because the fetal head cannot easily enter the lower segment. It occurs in about 1 in 200 pregnancies and is more common with twins (larger placenta), multiparity, increasing age, and previous caesarean section. After a bleed the uterus remains soft and the fetal heart is usually present.

Types of praevia
- major: Type III or IV – covers os partially or completely
- minor: Type I or II – just enters lower segment or reaches to edge of cervical os

Management
- admit (use paramedical ambulance service, never perform VE)
- resuscitate (i.v. infusion, saline or plasma expander, e.g. Haemaccel, or O-negative blood if urgent. Crossmatch blood)
- ascertain fetal viability/well-being
- ultrasound scan (to confirm diagnosis)
- if heavy bleeding persists – emergency section
- bleeding usually settles: the woman is kept in hospital, sometimes for the rest of the pregnancy. Re-scan may confirm persistent praevia (L/segment expands as third trimester advances) and also checks for IUGR which is more common due to the poor placental

site. Bedrest is not necessary. Blood is kept crossmatched and repeated transfusion can prolong the pregnancy if bleeding slight and recurrent. Check Hb freqently, give Fe and folate and chart fetal growth by USS. CTGs are important if there is further bleeding or IUGR. Give anti-D and check Kleihauer if Rhesus-negative.

Note: Caesarean section for placenta praevia is a technically difficult operation – abnormal fetal lie, haemorrhage, poor uterine contractility leading to increased PPH. Regional anaesthesia is contraindicated (poor vascular reflexes in lower limbs cannot compensate for major haemorrhage), and GA can be complex if there is severe haemorrhage. Consultant obstetrician (and senior anaesthetist) should attend theatre.

A low placenta on an earlier scan (e.g. 20 weeks) is not always a problem as later lower-segment formation allows the presenting part to pass the lower placental edge: repeat scans are indicated. **Note**: USS can miss partial placenta praevia, so never dismiss the possibility even if scan does not confirm, e.g. succenturiate lobe or lateral 'tongue' of placenta may not be seen.

If doubt exists, an EUA or examination in theatre (EIT) can be performed followed by immediate section if the placenta is indeed covering the os. If the placenta is low but not covering the os (type I or II praevia) labour can be induced by ARM and Syntocinon, with fetal monitoring.

Placental abruption

Typically the woman has sudden abdominal pain and becomes shocked with a hard tender uterus (retroplacental blood tracks into the myometrium) and absent fetal heart. Vaginal bleeding usually occurs (but haemorrhage may be concealed). It is wise to assume *under*estimation of loss in all cases. It can follow severe trauma (e.g. RTA) and is more common with severe IUGR/pre-eclampsia and with acute hydramnios.

Proteinuria is nearly always present.

Management

- resuscitate: wide bore cannula, i.v. infusion, CVP line, crossmatch blood (at least 4 units)
- opiate analgesia
- if the fetal heart is still present – deliver when condition stable (usually by caesarean section but if CTG normal and well advanced in labour, usually deliver easily vaginally after abruption)

Usually contractions have started, the head is engaged and the cervix is dilating. The membranes are ruptured, i.v. Syntocinon started and delivery usually occurs without delay.

Postpartum haemorrhage is the main risk and is often severe because the bruised uterus fails to contract properly and DIC occurs (due to thromboplastins: low fibrinogen and platelets; raised FDPs). Management involves ergometrine followed by syntocinon infusion and in the worst cases, intramyometrial $PGF_{2\alpha}$ (Hemabate). Sometimes bimanual compression or packing of the uterus in theatre is necessary. Use fresh-blood transfusion or fresh frozen plasma if possible to correct coagulopathy. Monitor urine output and CVP, since acute renal failure can follow (see page 169).

Marginal haemorrhage   Treat as for minor abruption. Quite often a woman has a painless bleed but the ultrasound scan shows a normally-situated placenta and speculum examination shows a normal cervix.

The bleeding is assumed to have come from the margin of the placenta. Admit for observation, crossmatch blood, monitor fetus. Provided it was not heavy, settles on bedrest and does not recur, the woman is allowed home (after anti-D if Rhesus-negative). The pregnancy is regarded as high-risk because these bleeds seem to be associated with increased PNM and the pregnancy should be monitored closely until delivery which may be electively preterm.

Incidental bleeds   Check cervix (take smear). Must exclude other causes by full investigation before making this diagnosis.

◆ Abdominal pain in pregnancy

a) *Uterine*
- miscarriage/preterm labour/ectopic
- abruption
- degeneration of fibroid
- uterine rupture

b) *Other gynaecological causes*
- ovarian cysts (especially rupture or torsion of dermoid)

c) *Non-gynaecological causes*
- renal (UTI, pyelitis, stones)
- gallstones
- appendicitis
- Meckel's diverticulum
- other rare causes (liver/gut/herniae)

Notes   1. *Pain in early pregnancy* is usually due to a threatened miscarriage. Pain that precedes bleeding suggests an ectopic. A retroverted uterus that fails to correct is rare but can become impacted in the pelvis (incarcerate) and causes urinary retention at about 14 weeks.

2. *In later pregnancy* the important point is whether or not the pain and tenderness is uterine. In *red degeneration* the woman is usually older and may be known to have fibroids from a previous scan. There can be fever and vomiting. If she rolls on her side the tender spot moves with the uterus. Treat with analgesics but avoid surgery.

In *abruption* the whole uterus is hard and tender, the woman is shocked and the fetal heart is usually lost. Resuscitate and deliver.

Rupture of a uterine scar can occur relatively silently in late pregnancy with gradually increasing pain and, later, shock. In early labour this is suspected if pain persists between contractions – contractions then cease. Laparotomy is necessary. Rupture is usually from a previous caesarean section (more risk if upper-segment or 'classical') or from a previous myomectomy or uterine perforations (rare but can happen).

3. *Ovarian cysts* are more likely to undergo torsion during pregnancy or the early puerperium. Pain severe but intermittent, with fever and leucocytosis.

4. *Appendicitis* is difficult to diagnose in pregnancy. Tenderness tends to move towards the loin from 14 weeks. Pressure in the right upper quadrant may produce pain in the RIF. There may be tenderness PR. Other 'gut' causes of pain occur rarely (peptic ulcer, cholecystitis, pancreatitis, obstruction). Inflammatory bowel disease can present for the first time in pregnancy.

5. *Pyelonephritis* occurs more frequently in pregnancy because the ureters are dilated. Fever, loin tenderness, dysuria and pyuria usually make the diagnosis obvious. Send an urgent MSU for culture and start i.v. Augmentin. Ultrasound is good at detecting renal obstruction (stones, hydronephrosis) and safe in pregnancy. Analgesics and antispasmodics are given and surgery avoided if possible. Recurrent UTIs warrant antibiotic prophylaxis for the rest of the pregnancy.

6. *Rare causes*. Pregnancy ileus is due to severe constipation and colonic dilation and is treated by 'drip and suck' and enemas.

Pregnancy can precipitate *porphyria* and urinary porphobilinogen should be checked if there are also psychiatric or neurological symptoms.

7. *X-rays* should be avoided in early pregnancy whenever possible. 5 rad in the first 12 weeks is associated with a $5\times$ increase in childhood malignancy – particularly the leukaemias.

Note: It is worthwhile remembering that laparotomy with ritodrine cover is much less likely to precipitate premature labour than prolonged fever and toxicity.

◆ Hydatidiform mole

Rare: incidence is approximately 1 : 1000 live births in UK. Can occur at any age but more common over 40 years. An abnormal cystic proliferation of the trophoblast, hence the characteristically high urinary HCG levels, hyperemesis and bilateral theca lutein cysts. There are two types:
– complete: no fetus at any stage
– partial: evidence of a fetus (but not usually viable)

Most often diagnosed on an early dating scan now.

The features are:
– large for dates (the uterus feels 'doughy', not cystic)
– vaginal bleeding $\pm$ vesicles
– early PET (hypertension, proteinuria)
– extremely high HCG levels
– 'snowstorm' on scan
– thyrotoxicosis (rare: HCG resembles TSH)

Management Measure HCG levels in *blood,* crossmatch blood for surgery, and do a chest X-ray before suction evacuation of the uterus with Syntocinon cover.

Careful histology and serial HCG measurement is necessary with long-term follow-up at one of the three specialist UK centres for HCG measurements (e.g. Charing Cross Hospital, London). Serum HCG must be checked every 2 weeks until normal and the patient then sends urine samples as requested, monthly, directly to the centre to check levels remain normal. Serum samples must be recommenced if urinary HCGs rise again.

Follow-up is for 6 months if the HCG is normal within 8 weeks of evacuation: pregnancy need not be delayed further. If HCG was *not* normal within 8 weeks, follow-up for 2 years. If the patient wishes a pregnancy before the 2 years are up, this may be reasonable if the HCG has settled for 6 months or more – the risk of subsequent chori-ocarcinoma in this group is 1 : 286. Send urine at 6 and 12 weeks after any subsequent pregnancy (whatever its outcome).

These women should always avoid conception for 6 months after HCG reaches normal levels. The chance of another mole is 1 : 75. Use of the sheath is recommended as O/C contraindicated until HCG has been normal for 6 months. Hormonal preparations (O/C or others) taken between evacuation and the time when HCG levels become normal increase the risk of development of invasive mole or chorio-carcinoma.

If HCG levels *rise* at any time after the first 8 weeks of follow-up, chemotherapy is indicated as for choriocarcinoma.

Choriocarcinoma. About 10% of moles are malignant. Risk of pro-gression to malignancy can be predicted using the blood group of the woman and her partner, age, and the nature of the preceding pregnancy (viable, miscarried, molar, etc.). It can occur after apparently normal pregnancies in which case it presents as irregular bleeding, anaemia and weight loss and is diagnosed on curettings. Chest X-ray may show metastases (lung and intracerebral are common sites), but early treat-ment with high-dose methotrexate cures almost 100%. Combination chemotherapy is used for high-risk cases or aggressive disease.

◆ Hyperemesis gravidarum

Nausea is common in pregnancy up to 16 weeks, possibly due to high HCG levels (reassure and observe) and may reappear near term.

Management of persistent vomiting

1. Dietary advice (small frequent meals, e.g. dry toast before rising, no tea/coffee and avoid fatty foods) and an anti-emetic, e.g. prochlorperazine. Acupressure (C-bands) or acupuncture may help.
2. Admit if prolonged or dehydrated and ketotic. Intravenous fluids (normal saline) are given and serum electrolytes monitored. Prolonged vomiting can cause proteinuria, jaundice and neuropa-thy (due to thiamine deficiency) – prescribe thiamine orally to pre-vent Wernicke's encephalopathy. Sedatives and anti-emetics are less teratogenic than prolonged ketosis.
3. Always exclude a UTI. Scan to exclude twins or a mole. If vomit-ing persists *consider other causes*:
   – abdomen (appendix, obstruction, twisted ovarian cyst)
   – raised intracranial pressure
   – metabolic (diabetes, hypercalcaemia)
4. Very rarely, termination is necessary for life-threatening dehydra-tion and ketosis.

5. In a prospective study of more than 16 000 women there was no difference in the incidence of congenital defects between those who had vomited in pregnancy and those who had not.
6. Nausea in later pregnancy can be due to reflux oesophagitis and responds to antacids.

◆ Twins

1 in 80 pregnancies. It may be suspected if there is a family history or a history of induced ovulation with clomiphene or gonadotrophins, or excessive hyperemesis, or if PET develops in a multip. Now almost always first diagnosed at the dating scan.

Clinically, the patient is large for dates, with three poles palpable and the diagnosis is confirmed by scan.

THE MAIN DANGER IS PREMATURE LABOUR. Book into a unit with a SCBU. Strict antenatal supervision is necessary to prevent anaemia or failure to recognise the onset of pre-eclampsia. Monitor the Hb regularly, give iron and folate supplements and admit early if hypertension occurs. UTI and acute pyelonephritis are more common with twins. Maternal weight gain is increased by about 4 kg (e.g. 14–16 kg). Do serial ultrasounds, at 20 weeks for anomaly, and then for growth (praevia, malpresentations and abnormal lie are also more common). Serum screening for Down's syndrome is inappropriate: individual assessment of each twin can be done by nuchal translucency scan but management dilemmas occur when one twin is affected and one not and careful counselling is required.

The early scan can identify accurately the nature of the membrane (if not mono-amniotic) between the two sacs. Mono-amniotic twins are at much greater risk from twin–twin transfusion (twin reversed arterial perfusion sequence or 'TRAP' – where one twin grows at the expense of the other) and should be referred to specialist units. Delivery is always more problematic also – caesarean section preferred. Most assisted-pregnancy multiple conceptions will be from separate oocytes (i.e. non-identical).

Twins often deliver spontaneously by 38 weeks but, if monitoring is satisfactory, may go to term quite safely. In labour both twins are monitored (the first by scalp electrode, the second externally). Epidural is recommended because operative intervention may be needed for the second twin, which is the one more at risk. Provided both twins have grown well and at least the first is cephalic, vaginal delivery can be advised.

After delivery of the first twin, it is particularly important to double-clamp the cord in the normal way in case the fetal circulations are connected by a placental anastomosis, when the second twin could exsanguinate (also avoid delay in delivery of second twin).

The assistant turns the lie of the second twin (abdominally) to longitudinal, while the vaginal operator checks the presenting part. When the presenting part descends into the pelvis, rupture the membranes and await delivery (if necessary start Syntocinon since contractions often tail off). The second twin is more at risk of hypoxia than the first and harder to assess. Ventouse or forceps (or traction on the legs if breech) should be used if there is any delay. Internal version (putting a hand into the uterus and pulling a leg down) is still sometimes used in this situation for cord prolapse or if the second twin remains transverse. Caesarean for the second twin is sometimes appropriate. There should be less than 20 minutes between vaginal deliveries of the first and second twins.

PPH is more likely: blood should have been crossmatched and i.v. ergometrine may be necessary.

Note: If the membrane separating the babies has only two layers (amnion but no chorion) the twins are monozygotic (identical).

Breastfeeding should be encouraged with twins.

◆ Breech

25% at 30 weeks but only 3% at term. Perinatal mortality is increased (cord prolapse, intracranial haemorrhage, congenital anomaly).

Diagnosed by:
- subcostal tenderness
- ballottable head
- (FH higher than usual)
- softer mass in pelvis
- VE – breech palpable through fornix (in labour identify by sacrum, anus or feet)
- ultrasound

Breech may be due to an abnormal uterine shape (e.g. bicornuate), praevia, pelvic mass (e.g. cyst) or to fetal anomaly.

Management
1. *Observe until 36 weeks* as it may well turn spontaneously.
2. *At 36 weeks refer for specialist opinion*, for scan and VE. Radiological pelvimetry (CT) is no longer felt to be of value

   Ultrasound scan excludes placenta praevia (or rarely hydrocephalus), confirms the diagnosis, measures the BPD, checks the position of the legs (extended legs safest (85% cases), footling breech carries a high risk of cord prolapse) and allows an estimate of fetal weight.

   VE confirms the diagnosis (which can be difficult in a primip with a deeply engaged breech) and excludes fibroids or an ovarian tumour. Clinical assessment of the size of the pelvic cavity is notoriously inaccurate.
3. *External cephalic version* is sometimes attempted if a vaginal delivery is being considered.

   It must be performed only by a skilled obstetrician and only if the uterus is lax and the breech easily moved. It should be performed gently and should be painless. The success rate even in experienced hands is only around 50%.

   There is a risk of placental separation or cord accident. Give anti-D if Rhesus negative.

   ECV is contraindicated if:
   - hypertensive
   - previous APH

  – uterine scar
  – caesarean planned anyway
4. *Elective section* is becoming increasingly common for breech presentations because of the higher PNM associated with vaginal breech deliveries.

  Some specialists choose C/S for all cases, others only if there is another complication (e.g. elderly primip, bad obstetric history, likely small pelvis, pre-eclampsia, diabetic).
5. *Vaginal delivery*. Spontaneous labour is preferred as it is more efficient (efficiency outweighs addition of fetal weight gain in last 2 weeks of pregnancy). Syntocinon only used with close supervision as delay in labour may indicate borderline pelvic diameters. Continuous monitoring mandatory. Early recourse to caesarean section for complications. Epidural recommended to avoid pushing before there is full dilatation and to permit easy operative intervention.
  – the bitrochanteric diameter engages in the AP position and the trunk is born by lateral flexion
  – elective episiotomy
  – traction in the groin may be needed to assist with flexion of knees. Abdominal traction on fetus to be avoided at all costs
  – if the arms become extended they are delivered by Løvset's manoeuvre (rotating a shoulder posteriorly then anteriorly again brings them down to be just under the pubic arch from where the arm can be brought down by an examining finger)
  – once the shoulders are delivered, the head is rotated to become AP (with the back upwards) and is delivered with forceps to guard the after coming head (safer for the cervical spine than the Mauriceau-Smellie-Veit manoeuvre)
  – paediatrician aspirates the baby's mouth before head delivery. Keep the body warm as baby cools a lot during delivery

◆ Unstable lie

An oblique or transverse lie is quite common before 36 weeks, especially in multiple pregnancies or with hydramnios. If it occurs after 37 weeks the patient should be admitted because of the danger of premature rupture of the membranes with cord prolapse. Only if it is neglected can impacted shoulder, obstructed labour and uterine rupture occur.

Management
1. Ultrasound scan (?placenta praevia).
2. Vaginal examination (?ovarian cyst, large fibroid).
3. Admit at 37 weeks and await labour. Crossmatch blood (increasing uterine activity makes SROM and cord prolapse a possibility).
(4. Some perform daily version, using the rationale that a stable lie becomes more likely as the fetus gets bigger and the volume of liquor falls from about 1 litre at 36 weeks to 500 ml at term. Rare nowadays as caesarean section has become a safer option.)
5. If the membranes rupture, VE to exclude cord prolapse.
6. If labour starts, correct the lie. If this is not possible C/S is performed.

7. After term a stabilising induction may be performed. A Syntocinon drip is started and the head held in the pelvis by one operator while another ruptures the membranes. Facilities for section must be ready in case of cord prolapse. The patient is kept in bed until the head is well engaged.

Note: A persistent abnormal lie suggests a uterine abnormality. (Bicornuate uterus is extremely difficult to diagnose on late USS.)

◆ Hydramnios

Amniotic fluid normally reaches a maximum volume of 1–1.5 litres at 36 weeks. It is produced from the placental amnion and fetal urine (and has the same biochemical composition as fetal urine) and is continuously being swallowed by the fetus.

Hydramnios means excessive liquor, usually from 32 weeks. It can cause pressure symptoms (dyspnoea, heartburn, oedema or postural hypotension due to IVC compression) and is associated with a high PNM (fetal abnormality, premature labour, cord prolapse, malpresentation).

Diagnosis:
- large-for-dates
- fluid thrill
- fetal parts difficult to feel
- fetal ballottement
- unstable lie
- ultrasound

Management
1. Exclude diabetes (test urine, timed random sugar, GLT or GTT), twins and anencephaly. Scan also excludes large ovarian cyst.
2. If there is discomfort, consider bedrest. Repeat amniocentesis to remove fluid if possible, but it reaccumulates rapidly and because this procedure increases the risks of infection and preterm delivery it is rarely done. Oral indometacin brings about changes in the fetal renal function (oliguria) and can temporarily reduce acute hydramnios: it cannot be used long term (risks of affecting fetal circulation through the ductus).
3. Consider induction for severe discomfort or fetal abnormality. Before induction, controlled, slow release of fluid by amniocentesis can reduce the rush of fluid and the risk of placental separation, but facilities for section should be prepared. PPH is more common.
4. The paediatrician may pass a nasogastric tube into the stomach of the infant after delivery to exclude oesophageal atresia.

◆ Preterm spontaneous rupture of the membranes

Without intervention, the membranes usually rupture late in labour. In about 8% of pregnancies the membranes rupture prematurely (i.e. before labour starts), but near to term, labour usually soon follows.

In 2% the membranes rupture before 37 weeks (preterm). The cause is usually unknown (a few cases are due to cervical incompetence,

hydramnios or trauma). *There are three problems*:
- possible cord prolapse (rare)
- ascending infection
- premature labour

Cord prolapse

In the rare event that a midwife or doctor is present when the membranes rupture, and particularly if there is a malpresentation (oblique lie or breech), a sterile VE should be performed to exclude cord prolapse.

If the cord is felt and is still pulsating (or if in any doubt), replace in the vagina (more easily done if it is wrapped in sterile gauze) and keep two fingers in the vagina, with upward pressure on the presenting part (until the woman can be delivered by section). Tip her head-down or use the knee–chest position. Call emergency paramedical ambulance.

Usually the woman is admitted unexamined because strict asepsis is necessary.

Diagnosis

Diagnosis is based on the history and examination with a sterile speculum (not digitally) revealing liquor (with its characteristic odour) running from the cervix. The pool of liquid in the vagina is diagnostic. False-positive results from Amnistix (nitrazine) are common.

Quite commonly the diagnosis is in doubt. The woman describes an intermittent trickle but no liquor is seen.

If sterile VE reveals intact membranes, the liquor was probably coming from a *hindwater leak*, and these generally seal spontaneously. Admit for observation, monitor the fetus, and allow home after a few days if there is no more fluid. Scan may be of some value.

If the problem is recurrent (?liquor, ?urine) a 200 mg tablet of Pyridium is occasionally used to stain the urine red.

Management

This now tends to be conservative (i.e. admit and await events) because recent studies have shown that most neonatal deaths are due to prematurity rather than infection. Prophylactic antibiotics are not helpful because they do not prevent infection in the neonate. However, the ORACLE trial (Overview of the Role of Antibiotics in prevention or Curtailing of preterm Labour) is still ongoing, aiming to assess whether antibiotics are of any value.
- admit for observation
- monitor the fetus
- group and reserve serum (in case of fetal distress and the need for emergency section)
- scan for estimated fetal weight, presentation and residual liquor volume. Preterm rupture of the membranes is said to be associated with fetal abnormality
- single HVS on admission (or send liquor for culture). Treat if proven infection but the efficacy of prophylaxis with negative microbiology is unproven and it may compromise paediatric assessment. Can repeat weekly (low vaginal swab as reliable as high vaginal swab and avoids repeat VEs)
- if signs of infection develop with fever, tachycardia and discharge, the baby has to be delivered (induction or section). A raised

C-reactive protein level may be a useful early indicator of infection (useful to check CRP weekly)

- once labour starts (usually within 7 days) it is allowed to proceed. Some advocate trying to delay labour for 24 hours with ritodrine so that steroids can be given to increase fetal surfactant levels (there is no evidence that steroids increase the infection rate)
- before 32 weeks the baby is usually delivered by C/S to decrease the risk of birth trauma to the premature infant (take paediatric advice)

◆ Premature labour

1. Defined as labour before 37 completed weeks. It tends to recur in subsequent pregnancies. About 2% of deliveries occur before 34 weeks and with modern SCBU facilities >95% of babies born at 32 weeks now survive and about 80% of those born at 26 weeks, although longer-term handicap can be a greater problem if extremely preterm.

2. Admit the woman to a unit with a SCBU – transfer *in utero* is safer than post-delivery transfer in an incubator. Attempts to stop labour are most effective when started early so IF IN DOUBT – REFER.

3. VE to assess cervical dilatation. If the cervix is 4 cm or more, or the membranes rupture, labour is allowed to continue. Sometimes painful contractions occur without cervical dilatation.

4. Always check an MSU and treat if infected. Often no cause is found but it may be due to UTI (which can be asymptomatic), high fever, twins, hydramnios, abruption or cervical incompetence.

5. After 34 weeks, labour is allowed to proceed (very rarely, if gestation is in doubt, L : S ratio may be indicated). Before 34 weeks, if membranes are intact, an intravenous infusion of a β-sympathomimetic can be started, e.g. ritodrine (Yutopar) starting at 50 µg/min increasing to 400 µg/min. Use syringe pump to reduce fluid volume required. Evidence of benefit is shown in terms of delaying delivery, but no improvement in perinatal mortality has been demonstrated.

   This suppresses labour in about 80% of cases if cervical dilatation is still <2 cm. Side-effects of tachycardia, palpitations, tremor and feelings of panic can occur. Salbutamol is also effective.

6. If labour is not suppressed, prompt delivery is the aim, although some advocate 48 hours delay, if possible, so dexamethasone 8 mg × 2 doses or betamethasone 12 mg × 2 doses can be given to decrease the chance of RDS. The combination of sympathomimetics and steroids can be dangerous (cardiac failure and fluid overload) and maternal deaths have been recorded.

   Before 32 weeks caesarean section is often performed to avoid birth trauma. For vaginal delivery, epidural is helpful (to avoid opiates) and elective episiotomy to avoid birth trauma, with full intrapartum monitoring and a paediatrician present at the delivery.

7. Premature labour tends to recur in subsequent pregnancies. A hysterosalpingogram may be indicated if cervical incompetence is suspected, so that a cervical suture can be inserted in the next pregnancy.

During antenatal care, a digital examination can be performed at each visit in order to detect cervical incompetence if there is a history of termination or premature labour. Reliability is uncertain, however. Usually go on history, but TV scanning can help in assessment.

◆ Postmaturity

1. About 10% of pregnancies reach 42 weeks. PNM rises after this due to placental insufficiency and probably because the fetal head is larger, harder and moulds less easily. The incidence of fetal distress in labour is higher.
2. *Why is labour delayed?* The maturing fetal adrenal seems to initiate labour (and cortisol also stimulates surfactant production) and it may be that the fetus is not yet 'ready' to deliver. Sometimes gestation is not certain, when it is difficult to be sure that the pregnancy is postmature.
3. From 40 weeks the fetus can be monitored by a kick chart. Labour is not usually induced until 42 weeks unless there is another complication (e.g. hypertension). Before induction the dates should be checked and the cervix should be favourable. The fetus is monitored in labour and fetal distress in labour is an indication for section.
4. Induced labour is less efficient – primips induced at 42 weeks have an increased chance of failed induction or poor progress in the first stage, and oxytocics must be administered with caution in multips.

◆ Home deliveries

Between 1950 and 1990 the number of women having their baby in hospital increased in some areas from 50 to 98%. Since 1950 the PNM has fallen from 35 to 7 – more due to improvements in general health and nutrition than the place of delivery.

There has been a recent trend back to wanting home deliveries. Some of *the reasons* are:
– dislike of hospital environment
– bad previous experience (self or a friend)
– other children at home
– cost of travel
– statistics from other countries, e.g. The Netherlands, consistently show a majority of home births and yet their PNM is lower than that for the UK.

The *safety* of home births is a complex issue and has a lot to do with expectation, professional training and independence, and many other factors. The safety of the mother, not just her baby, must be considered in making the correct choice.

If a woman requests a home delivery, the GP should discuss her reasons and point out *the alternatives*:
– 'DOMINO' delivery, with her own district midwife delivering her in the consultant unit

- 6-hour discharge
- early transfer to GP unit nearer home

If a home delivery is planned there should be good, shared antenatal care so that the GP, midwife and health visitor can assess suitability for home confinement. The community team must know the woman and assess the suitability of her home (heating, lighting, hygiene, telephone, accessibility, additional help).

Both the midwife and the GP, or two midwives, must be present at a home delivery because the mother and baby may need attention at the same time. They must be competent at resuscitation of the newborn and must keep intubation technique up to date. 7% of low-risk pregnancies produce life-threatening situations (neonatal asphyxia, postpartum haemorrhage).

Planned home confinement requires strict criteria for safety. The couple must be aware of the slightly increased risk (probably 1/1000 increase in PNM) and that there is a 1 in 5 chance of needing transfer for hospital delivery for reasons detected antenatally (15%) or in labour (5%).

The woman must be carefully selected. The following should be *excluded*:

- parity above 4 (risk of PPH)
- poor home conditions
- bad obstetric history. Previous operative delivery/PPH/manual removal of placenta
- previous low birth weight baby
- medical conditions (diabetes, heart disease)
- gynaecological operations (myomectomy, cone biopsy)
- APH

The GP must be competent (including neonatal intubation) *and available* (or have an equally competent named deputy to cover off-duty periods) and fully equipped. There must be easy access to hospital facilities and an obstetric/paramedic emergency service must be available. The role of the GP is largely supervisory. Careful selection and monitoring of patients antenatally makes emergencies rare, but nevertheless GP must be prepared.

Equipment Equipment for home confinement (packs usually supplied by the district midwife) includes:

- sterile packs
  - a) maternity pack
  - b) vaginal examination pack
  - c) delivery pack
  - d) baby pack
  - c) repair pack
- sphygmomanometer and thermometer
- fetal stethoscope (sonicaid amplifier ideally)
- Entonox machine
- Amnihook (Hollister)
- Wrigley's forceps or hand-held ventouse
- infant laryngoscope, tracheal tube, sucker
- episiotomy scissors

- sutures (dexon or vicryl)
- urine testing equipment
- blood collection equipment
- i.v. giving set. Dextrose saline (Haemaccel)
- drugs (check expiry dates)
  a) pethidine
  b) naloxone
  c) syntometrine
  d) lignocaine (2%)
  e) diazepam
  f) hydralazine

Good antenatal care reduces the risk of home confinement. Routine antenatal care is as normal. The GP is notified at the onset of labour, and must attend early because this improves assessment later if the patient needs transfer to a consultant unit.

Indications for hospital transfer

Conditions indicating transfer are:
- premature labour
- delay in 1st stage (24 hours primip, 12 hours multip)
- delay in 2nd stage (or failure to progress)
- bleeding early in labour
- fetal distress (assess fetal heart rate, meconium staining)
- cord prolapse (1 in 2000 low-risk pregnancies)

Postdelivery, a retained placenta and PPH are indications for urgent transfer with supervision. Following normal deliveries 6% of babies require assistance with breathing and the GP must be competent at this. Unexpected PPH or birth asphyxia are the main hazards in home confinement.

◆ Documentation in pregnancy

1. Form FP24 (doctor's *claim for payment* for maternity services) must be signed by the patient at booking. Part 3 is filled in at the 6-week postnatal and sent to the FPA.
2. Form FW8 (*certificate of pregnancy*) must be completed by the woman, signed by the doctor (or midwife) and sent to the FPA. It entitles her to free prescriptions, dental treatment and milk.
3. Maternity *booking form* – filled in by the GP (or midwife) and sent to the hospital to book the delivery. It states the length of stay that the doctor or midwife feels is appropriate, having visited the home. Copies are sent to:
   - the maternity hospital
   - district midwife
   - health visitor
   - GP
4. Form MatB1 (*certificate of expected confinement*) – must be signed by the GP (or midwife) at 26 weeks. The woman sends this to the DoH to claim for maternity benefits.
5. Cooperation card (or hand-held notes) – kept by the patient and now used by many hospitals.

◆ Induction of labour

Indications
- conditions associated with placental insufficiency, if fetal monitoring suggests chronic hypoxia (IUGR, APH, postmaturity)
- conditions with a known risk to the fetus (diabetes, Rhesus disease)
- fetal death or abnormality (if appropriate for TOP or for specialised paediatric involvement at predetermined time)
- risk to the mother (PET, abruption)

Social reasons for induction include imminent family bereavement (e.g. grandparent), partner overseas, etc. But social IOL needs to be discussed at length to ensure that the couple understand the increased risks (of the need for caesarean section, prematurity, etc.).

Note: It is *essential* to be certain of gestation before induction.

Method
The classical method of inducing labour is a combination of amniotomy and i.v. Syntocinon infusion. Induction by prostaglandin p.v. (1 or 2 mg gel best) if Bishop score of cervix is poor is preferable to ARM and Syntocinon in most cases. If the cervix is unfavourable repeated PG doses may be used to 'soften' the cervix prior to ARM. PG may cause hypertonic contraction and should be used with caution in grand multips, IUGR, previous caesarean section, etc. Induction is likely to fail if the cervix is not favourable (especially in a primip) and the woman may then have to be delivered by section. If the membranes have been ruptured for more than 24 hours there is a risk of infection.

Induction is obviously contraindicated if there is disproportion (e.g. pelvic tumour, transverse lie).

Assessment
The cervix must be assessed. Signs that the cervix is *favourable* for induction are:
- well-effaced (i.e. shortened)
- dilated 2 cm or more
- anterior (and easy to reach)
- soft
- head well engaged (i.e. the whole of the fetal head below the level of the pubis on palpation; the head 2 cm or less above the ischial spines on VE)

If these signs are all favourable, induction is very likely to succeed.

Induction is more likely to fail if the cervix is *unfavourable*:
- long (e.g. 2 cm)
- closed (does not admit a finger)
- posterior (and difficult to palpate)
- firm

The *Bishop score*, or now the modified or 'Calder' score, is sometimes used as a guide to the ripeness of the cervix for induction. Each of the five signs is scored (1, 2 or 3) and a score above 7 (maximum 13) means that induction is more likely to succeed.

If the cervix is unfavourable, prostaglandin E_2 (Prostin) in tylose gel is delivered into the posterior fornix and usually causes ripening of the cervix over 24 hours. Sometimes it even induces labour; sometimes it needs to be repeated. Misoprostol (oral or vaginal tablets) is an alternative used in some units.

Management
- explain and consent verbally
- check the gestation
- confirm the presentation
- sterile VE to assess the cervix. Sweep the membranes and stretch the cervix (this releases prostaglandins and encourages contractions to start). Rupture the forewaters if the findings are favourable (usually > 4 cm) with an amniotomy hook (e.g. plastic Amnihook). Exclude cord prolapse
- note colour and volume of liquor. Bleeding suggests ruptured vasa praevia (blood contains HbF if fetal, HbA if maternal) and, together with fetal distress, is an indication for immediate section
- apply a fetal scalp electrode (FSE) if continuous electronic monitoring is required (with permission) and start continuous CTG monitoring (otherwise check the fetal heart by auscultation or monitor externally)
- record the findings in the notes. Begin partogram. Mobilise if possible
- in a primip i.v. Syntocinon infusion is usually only started after 2–3 hours if PG was used before, as PG and ARM is usually sufficient without Syntocinon. (Begin at 0.5–1 mU/minute via syringe pump, doubling every 20 minutes until regular contractions occur.) In a multip with a ripe cervix labour often starts after amniotomy with mobilisation: if Syntocinon is used start at very low doses. Once established, the Syntocinon rate can often be reduced.
- hyperstimulation must be avoided

◆ First stage of labour

This lasts from the onset of regular painful contractions to full dilatation of the cervix (10 cm).

The woman often telephones the labour ward and is admitted if she mentions:
- regular pains (e.g. every 10 minutes)
- show (mucus plug from cervix)
- blood (usually means a show)
- 'waters gone' (ruptured membranes)

The active management of labour means that prolonged labour, with increased risks of infection and fetal hypoxia, is no longer common.

The *aims* are:
- to monitor fetus, mother and progress
- to prevent pain and infection
- to augment labour if progress is slow

REMEMBER – as long as there is progressive cervical dilatation and the fetal condition is good, labour is normal; if abnormal, then the possibilities are either augmentation with Syntocinon or caesarean section.

Management
1. Admit, check antenatal notes (full history if none) and examine for lie, presentation, fetal heart and the state of the cervix.

2. Group and save serum and check Hb if:
   - anaemic
   - section is a possible outcome (PET, IUGR, APH, breech, unstable lie, uterine scar or previous long labour)
   - PPH is more likely (high parity, twins, hydramnios, previous PPH, fibroids or if labour becomes prolonged)
3. Perform short (20 minutes) 'admission CTG' to ascertain fetal state at outset. Refer for senior opinion unless entirely normal.
4. Discuss analgesia:
   - transcutaneous nerve stimulation
   - pethidine/Meptid
   - Entonox
   - epidural
   - (acupuncture, if pre-arranged, can be useful for some women)
5. The woman may bathe and is encouraged to walk about in the early stages. All urine is tested. She is allowed clear fluids only (in case urgent GA is necessary).
6. The midwife monitors (and records on partogram):
   - TPR
   - urinalysis (ketones, protein, glucose)
   - fetal heart rate
   - contraction strengh and frequency
   - cervical dilatation
   - liquor colour
   - drugs
7. *Maternal distress*, i.e. signs of dehydration, exhaustion or disorientation (tachycardia, oliguria, ketonuria), is treated with 5% dextrose infusion.
8. *Progress* is assessed by:
   - cervical dilatation
   - contractions (frequency, strength, duration)
   - descent of the head (abdominally and vaginally)

   Cervical dilatation is slower up to about 3–4 cm (latent phase) then more rapid (active phase), but as a guide should be at least 1 cm/hour (in active phase) for primips and multips.

   Contractions: initially occur roughly every 10 minutes and steadily increase to every 2–3 minutes in established labour. The frequency of contractions is usually recorded as the number per 10 minutes (e.g. '3 in 10'), each one lasting about a minute. The strength and duration are noted as well.

   Descent of the head is usually described in relation to the ischial spines (normally the head is 2 cm above spines when it is just engaged). However, ALWAYS PALPATE ABDOMINALLY because, with a lot of caput and moulding, a non-engaged head *can* be felt well below the spines.
9. VEs must be sterile. The vulva is cleaned each time (plain water or 1% chlorhexidine). Hibitane cream is used as a lubricant.

   VE is performed on admission (and the membranes are ruptured if labour is established, i.e. regular contractions and cervical dilatation, in order to exclude meconium-stained liquor). VE is also performed if the membranes rupture spontaneously (to exclude cord prolapse).

VEs are performed 2–4 hourly in labour to assess dilatation of the cervix and the position and descent of the head, and more frequently at the end of labour using the partogram when full dilatation should be achieved.

At each VE *record in the notes:*
- abdominal palpation in fifths palpable above the brim
- cervix (dilatation, effacement, ?well or poorly applied to the fetal head)
- presentation – vertex (rarely breech, brow, face)
- position of the occiput (usually LOT, then LOA, then OA as it descends)
- level of head (-3, -2, -1 cm above spines, at spines, or 1, 2, 3 cm below spines)
- membranes (intact or ruptured)
- no cord felt (cord prolapse needs emergency section if the baby is still alive)
- loss (meconium, blood, liquor, nil draining)

Delay in the first stage   The first stage normally takes approximately 12 hours in a primip and 6 hours in a multip.

'Active management' means that if progress is too slow, labour is augmented with Syntocinon – this decreases the complications of a long labour (fetal hypoxia, maternal acidosis, infection). Exclude contraindications prior to starting Syntocinon.

The rate of cervical dilatation recorded on a partogram is the most important method of assessing progress (frequency of contractions and descent of the head are also important). If labour falls behind the normal rate (approx. 1 cm/hour), then labour is augmented. Amniotomy is performed (if it has not been performed earlier) and i.v. Syntocinon started (1–4 mU/min) according to local guidelines until the contractions are strong and regular (every 2–3 minutes). Good contractions will overcome *minor* disproportion.

Note: Multips need closer supervision of Syntocinon because uterine rupture is a greater possibility.

Continuous fetal monitoring is essential whenever Syntocinon is used.

If 2–3 hours of good contractions fail to produce progress, with no further dilatation, thinning or effacement (shortening) of the cervix, then *cephalo–pelvic disproportion* is diagnosed. Often there is excessive caput and moulding of the fetal skull (and if neglected uterine rupture could occur) and section is indicated.

The concept of the active management of labour is largely due to O'Driscoll, who emphasises that the most important part of good management is the certain diagnosis of labour – BEFORE any intervention to augment it.

◆ Intrapartum monitoring

This is a type of *screening* for fetal distress – *diagnosis* would require fetal oxygenation and acid–base status assessment. The discovery of the relation between fetal acidosis and the fetal heart rate led to fetal monitoring in the 1970s. *The aim is the early diagnosis of intrapartum asphyxia.* A continuous CTG is recorded of the fetal heart rate via an external transducer or a scalp electrode, and of uterine contractions via an abdominal pressure transducer (or intrauterine catheter).

Indications:

1. Cases where fetal distress is more likely (e.g. IUGR, pre-eclampsia, diabetes, postmaturity).
2. Whenever labour is induced or augmented with i.v. Syntocinon.
3. If the liquor is meconium-stained – 10% have fetal distress (hypoxia causes gut motility and relaxation of sphincters).
4. With an epidural (maternal hypotension may cause bradycardia).

The *normal CTG* shows:
– rate 110–155
– good beat-to-beat (short term) variability (normally 5–10)
– accelerations (with palpation or fetal movements)

Signs of probable hypoxia are:
– flat trace (loss of short-term variability)
– tachycardia (rate above 160)
– bradycardia (rate below 110)
– early decelerations (with contractions)
– late decelerations (persisting after a contraction)
– variable deceleration (unassociated with contractions)

Combinations of these are more serious, e.g. a flat trace with a base-line tachycardia and early decelerations would indicate the need to take a fetal blood sample and in some situations (e.g. early labour or trial of labour) might be an indication for section.

Unprovoked deceleration in early labour may indicate section (the fetus is unlikely to tolerate the hypoxia of late labour contractions).

Early decelerations are common in the second stage of labour due to powerful contractions (deep ones sometimes occur if the cord is round the neck). As long as recovery is rapid after a contraction no action is needed.

The management of a poor CTG trace

1. Lie the woman on her side, stop Syntocinon and give oxygen (IVC compression causes maternal hypotension): uses the placenta to resuscitate the baby in utero. Often the trace returns to normal.
2. Exclude maternal ketosis or excessive contractions due to Syntocinon. Perform abdominal examination and VE.
3. Take a *fetal blood sample* (capillary blood from the fetal scalp). CTG is a *screening* method and only about 50% of cases with a poor CTG trace are actually hypoxic (and acidotic).

Management depends on blood pH:
above 7.3 – normal
7.2–7.3 – repeat
below 7.2 – emergency delivery (usually section)

Continuous CTG vs intermittent auscultation: A large trial in Dublin confirmed that the outcome in babies was similar for both the monitored groups. There were more neonatal convulsions in the group not using continuous electronic monitoring but no long-term sequelae were noted. There was more intervention (pH measurement, forceps or caesarean section) in the electronically monitored group. However, when considering such trial data it is important to remember that *all* forms of surveillance in labour rely on the *experience* of the supervising midwife/doctor in correctly interpreting the findings. A CTG trace incorrectly interpreted or interpreted in isolation from other findings (such as slow progress or meconium) is highly dangerous.

◆ Pain relief in labour

Pain in labour is due to:
- uterine ischaemia
- cervical dilatation (sacral pain)
- perineal stretching (pudendal nerve)

As the head presses on the pelvic floor, the woman pushes (by reflex action) and this often helps relieve the pain.

1. The woman must not be left alone in labour. *Understanding the events of labour* decreases pain. *Psychoprophylactic techniques*, for example those taught by the National Childbirth Trust, can be very helpful (used alone or with conventional analgesia). *Continuous care by a single named (and known) midwife* throughout greatly reduces the analgesic requirements of women in labour.

2. Early in labour, especially at night, a mild sedative is often requested but should be avoided. Two paracetamol tablets is a better alternative.

3. *Epidural* is indicated if there is hypertension, the likelihood of prolonged labour, forceps or section, or severe pain (usually in a primip).

   It should not be inserted until labour is established and ongoing (at least 3 cm dilated with good contractions).

   A needle is inserted between L1 and L2 (or into the sacral hiatus – a caudal block). The sensory fibres of the uterus go up to T11. A polythene catheter is threaded through the needle and is left in the epidural space so that repeated doses of local anaesthetic can be given, usually 0.25% bupivacaine (Marcain) approx. 10 ml every 2 hours. It can cause hypotension and BP must be carefully monitored after each dose. Hypotension is treated by lying the patient in the left lateral position and infusing 500 ml of Hartmann's solution. Spinal (i.e. subdural) injection can rarely cause phrenic nerve block and respiratory arrest and is therefore not practised. Analgesia is complete (although it can occasionally be unilateral) and the woman also loses sensation in the legs and bladder (examine regularly for bladder distension, which prevents descent of the head, and catheterise if necessary). Epidural anaesthesia prevents pushing and increases the need for forceps × 10 but has no other ill-effects.

4. The alternative to an epidural is the use of pethidine, Meptid or diamorphine analgesia for the first stage with Entonox for the second stage, together with pudendal block if forceps are necessary.

Pethidine: a State Registered Midwife is allowed to give 100 mg twice during labour. The usual dose is 100–150 mg i.m. followed by 50–100 mg every 2 hours up to a maximum of 400 mg in labour. It may cause nausea and metoclopramide (Maxalon) 10 mg i.m. may be given with it. Dystonic reactions to metoclopramide are most common in young women and may be seen in the labour ward situation (oculogyric crises). Promazine is sometimes given as a sedative but it is a poor anti-emetic, is not analgesic, and should be discouraged. Patient controlled analgesia (PCA) can be helpful.

Pethidine is avoided if possible within 2 hours of delivery as it can cause respiratory depression in the newborn – reversible with naloxone (Narcan) 0.01 mg/kg. *Diamorphine* is no more of a respiratory depressant in equi-analgesic doses than pethidine and is a better analgesic for labour.

Inhalational analgesia is often used in the second stage. Entonox (50% nitrous oxide, 50% oxygen) is used. It takes 20–30 seconds to be effective and needs to be started at the very beginning of a contraction. It is not used between contractions.

5. *Transcutaneous nerve stimulation*. Pain relief is based upon Melzack's Gate Theory of pain. Stimulation of large, afferent 'A' nerve fibres should block smaller pain-carrying 'C' fibres from transmitting to the brain. This is achieved by applying a small, variable current through electrodes placed on either side of the lower thoracic and upper lumbar spine. The results have been equivocal, some women reporting benefit in the first stage of labour, but little or no benefit during the second stage. There have, however, been reports of an overall reduction in the need for pethidine in labour when the technique has been used. It seems to have no effect on the baby or on the duration of labour.

◆ Second stage of labour

This lasts from full dilatation of the cervix (10 cm) to delivery of the baby and should not last longer than an hour. Full dilatation is suspected once the women gets the reflex urge to bear down (as the fetal head presses on the pelvic floor). It is also suspected if:
– the anus shows dilatation
– perineum bulges
– bleed (vaginal tear)
– head is visible (?caput)

It is confirmed by VE (the cervix is no longer palpable).

Note: with a lot of caput the head may be visible before the cervix is fully dilated.

Preparations for delivery are started when the head is visible in a primip (or when reflex pushing starts in a multip). Sterile conditions are essential.
1. Rupture the membranes if still intact (rare nowadays).
2. Hold a sterile pad over the anus.
3. If episiotomy is necessary infiltrate the perineum with 1% lignocaine and make the cut at the height of a contraction.

4. When delivery of the head is imminent, pressure from the left hand is used to hold the head flexed and also to prevent sudden delivery of the head (causing cranial trauma and perineal tears).

5. When the head is crowned (i.e. the occiput has passed under the pubis) the woman is told to stop the pushing and pant and the head is allowed to extend slowly between the contractions. The perineum is pushed down over the baby's face with the sterile pad.

6. Feel for the cord round the baby's neck (30%) and slip it over the baby's head. If it is too tight cut it between two clamps (then don't wait!).

7. Wait for the external rotation of the head. Deliver the anterior shoulder with the next contraction by gently pulling the head down (towards the mother's sacrum) then upwards to deliver the posterior shoulder. If there is difficulty with the anterior shoulder (shoulder dystocia) ask the woman to push, ask an assistant to apply suprapubic pressure and if necessary put two fingers in the anterior axilla and pull down.

   Syntometrine i.m. is given with delivery of the anterior shoulder. (contains 5 units oxytocin + 0.5 mg ergometrine in 1 ml).

8. Suck out the baby's pharynx with a mucus extractor and clamp the cord. As soon as normal breathing is established, the baby should be dried and given to the mother, who can breastfeed immediately.

Delay in the second stage

The second stage is most usefully divided into two distinct phases: passive and active. The time spent in the active phase is of relevance when assessing fetal risk. Prolonged time spent in the passive phase may contribute to greater pudendal nerve damage to the mother.

The head engages in the wider transverse diameter of the pelvic *inlet* (transverse = 13 cm; AP = 11 cm). It descends onto the pelvic floor and then turns (*internal rotation*) so that the occiput turns forward and the widest diameter of the head now lies in the wider AP diameter of the *outlet* (AP = 13 cm; transverse = 11 cm). The head is born by extension of the baby's neck and the head then turns to the side (*external rotation*) because the shoulders are positioned in the AP diameter as they descend.

The second stage is normal if there is progressive descent of the head and the fetal condition remains good.

Causes

Delay may be due to:
- poor contractions
- poor maternal effort (pushing)
- failure of the head to rotate (OP, transverse)
- malpresentation (face, brow)
- outlet contracture (very rare)
- fetal ascites (very rare)
- abnormally large baby (diabetic mother)

10% of vertex deliveries are OP.

Poor contractions in the second stage are an unusual problem now because labour is augmented at an early stage if contractions are inadequate.

Table 6 Malpresentation

Palpation	Diagnosis	Presenting diameter and probable outcome
Posterior fontanelle (3 radiating sutures) Usually LOT then LOA then OA	Fully-flexed vertex	(Suboccipito-bregmatic) 9.5 cm Normal delivery
Anterior fontanelle (4 radiating sutures), is felt anteriorly Sometimes the posterior fontanelle is also palpable posteriorly	OP position, with poorly-flexed vertex (If in doubt which fontanelle is which, feel for an ear, which points to the occiput.) The anterior lip of the cervix is often oedematous	(Occipito-frontal) 11.5 cm Prolonged labour The head may eventually rotate to OA, or need to be rotated (with Keilland's or manually). Occasionally the head descends OP And delivers face-to-pubis
Anterior fontanelle and supra-orbital ridges	Brow (1 in 500) A high head may already have been noticed on abdominal examination	(Mento-vertical) 13.5 cm Obstructed labour and caesarean section
Softness (oedema) Bridge of nose, mouth	Face (1 in 300)	(Submento-bregmatic) 9.5 cm Mento-anterior will deliver. Mento-posterior obstructs and needs section

The most common cause of delay is an epidural causing anaesthesia of the pelvic floor with loss of the guttering effect of the levator ani, when the head remains in the transverse position.

VE is performed to determine the position. Sometimes *malpresentation*, especially brow, is not diagnosed until the second stage. Table 6 summarises the diagnosis and outcome of malpresentation.

Management The second stage is not usually allowed to last longer than 1 hour in a primip and about 30 minutes in a multip (although, with intrapartum monitoring, if the fetal condition is good and slow descent is occurring it is safe to continue). If an epidural is in place for the first stage, the head is usually allowed to descend for up to 1 hour (if observations satisfactory) before active pushing is commenced.

There may be marked caput and moulding but if the head is well engaged (examine abdominally) it will almost always be possible to deliver vaginally.

If the head has failed to rotate it may be possible to rotate the head manually to OA and then apply Neville-Barnes' forceps. Alternatively, Keilland's forceps or ventouse is used.

◆ Episiotomy

The *indications* for episiotomy are:
- tight perineum that is causing delay in the second stage (usually a primip), or threatened perineal tear
- forceps delivery or manual rotation. In a persistent OP position (born face-to-pubis), episiotomy is usually necessary because the larger occipito-frontal diameter is distending the vulva
- breech and premature deliveries to decrease trauma to the head
- fetal distress in the second stage (to hasten delivery)

The *complications* are:
1. Discomfort. Ice packs and analgesics help.
2. Haemorrhage. Vulvovaginal haematoma can cause severe pain and shock and needs to be drained and resutured under anaesthesic.
3. Infection.
4. Dyspareunia. Due to tight or malaligned repair which occasionally needs later surgery.
5. Rectovaginal fistula if rectum is sutured during repair (always perform a PR at the end of the procedure).
6. Damage to the anal sphincter (and faecal incontinence) due to extension of a midline episiotomy.

◆ Forceps

Forceps are *indicated* in:
- delay in the second stage
- fetal distress in the second stage
- elective (hypertension, heart disease or, rarely, intracranial problems such as subarachnoid haemorrhage)

There are two types:
1. Ventouse or low forceps (Neville-Barnes') if the head is OA.
2. Mid-cavity rotational forceps (Keilland's) if transverse or OP.

The left (mother's left) blade is always applied first. Ventouse or manual rotation (when possible) is safer than Keilland's rotation with less risk of skull fractures, intracranial haemorrhage and facial palsy. Forceps should never be applied to a high head (i.e. above the spines) – C/S is much safer.

The following conditions must be fulfilled:
- head engaged (per abdo), below spines per vaginam
- cervix fully dilated
- membranes ruptured
- good contractions
- empty bladder (always catheterise)
- pudendal block (or epidural)

- episiotomy
- (consent)

The pudendal nerve curves around the ischial spine. 10 ml of ligno-caine is infiltrated around each side (transvaginally or percuta-neously). This produces adequate vulval analgesia anteriorly but it is still necessary to infiltrate the perineum posteriorly.

◆ Vacuum extraction

The vacuum extractor, or ventouse, was designed by Malmström and introduced into Sweden in 1954.

The risk of trauma to the birth canal is less but the risk of cephalo-haematoma is increased when compared with forceps. It is particu-larly useful if the head is in the occipito-lateral position, as the head often rotates spontaneously during vacuum extraction. The mother can still bear down and assist with the delivery. It is safer than forceps in inexperienced hands.

It is contraindicated if the fetal head is high because prolonged extraction can cause fetal scalp necrosis. It is also contraindicated in preterm infants due to increased risk of haematoma (clotting defi-ciency in prematures).

◆ Caesarean section

Ideally this is performed under regional block (spinal or epidural) which entails fewer risks for the mother and has the advantage of immediate mother–infant contact.

The rate is about 15–18% in most UK units, and rising, due to higher numbers of section for 'fetal distress' diagnosed by CTG in labour, and to increasing use for breech and multiple pregnancy. Increasingly, parents may request elective caesarean section and should be counselled by a consultant. The maternal mortality is 1 per 10 000 for planned term C/S under regional block (which is 10 times that for vaginal delivery) due to complications of aspiration, pul-monary embolus, haemorrhage and infection.

The *recurring indications* are:
- cephalo–pelvic disproportion
- previous C/S
- previous successful incontinence procedure
- previous third-degree tear with successful outcome

The *non-recurring indications* for *elective section* are:
- placenta praevia or abruption
- pelvic cyst or fibroid
- severe PET
- some preterm situations
- placental insufficiency
- malpresentation (breech/transverse)

Indications for emergency section are:
- cord prolapse
- failure to progress in the first or second stage

- fetal distress in the first stage
- abruption/intrapartum haemorrhage (if fetus is still alive)
- transverse lie in labour

Note: Trial of labour may be allowed in subsequent pregnancy following one section, but most (not all) obstetricians recommend 'two sections, always a section'.

◆ Third stage of labour

This lasts from the delivery of the child to the delivery of the placenta (usually about 10 minutes). Without intervention, there is an interval of several minutes before contractions return, causing:

a) placental separation (and bleeding)
b) placental expulsion (allowing the uterus to contract and so clamp the maternal vessels feeding the placental site)

There is firm evidence that *active management* of the third stage decreases blood loss. Active management means:
- Syntometrine (to speed separation)
- controlled cord traction (to speed expulsion)

Syntometrine 1 ml i.m. is given with the delivery of the anterior shoulder. 1 ml Syntometrine contains 5 units of oxytocin (which acts rapidly to cause powerful regular contractions and speed placental separation) and 0.5 mg ergometrine (which causes sustained uterine spasm after 7 minutes, i.e. once the placenta is out, and lasts 1 hour). Once Syntometrine has been given do not wait for signs of placental separation before proceeding, or the placenta will be retained.

The *signs of placental separation* are:
- fundus rises and gets harder and rounder, cord lengthens
- pushing up on the uterus no longer retracts the cord
- gush of blood
- placenta visible, or palpable in the vagina

The placenta separates within minutes and *expulsion* is then hastened by controlled cord traction (the Brandt-Andrews technique). The essential part of this technique is simultaneous upward pressure on the uterus to prevent acute inversion of the uterus (see below), while steady tension is applied to the cord.

The placenta is delivered from the vagina by an up-and-down motion and blood loss is collected and measured. The fundus is massaged to expel any clots. A Syntocinon infusion (40 units in 500 ml) may be required for 1–2 hours to maintain the uterine contraction.

Complications   *Check the placenta.* There should be three vessels (two arteries, one vein) and the presence of only two vessels suggests that the baby may have renal or other abnormalities, but is usually normal.

If the placenta is incomplete, the uterus has to be explored immediately. Inspect the membrane. A hole in the chorion to which vessels pass suggests a succenturiate lobe has been retained. If pieces of membrane are retained they pass out in 2–3 days and usually no action is needed.

Continue to monitor BP every 30 minutes, especially if there is headache, visual disturbance or epigastric pain, as *postpartum hypertension and eclampsia can occur.*

Retained placenta If the placenta cannot be removed, crossmatch blood and start an i.v. infusion.

It is best then to wait about 30 minutes, provided there is no bleeding, because sometimes spasm of the cervix has trapped the separated placenta and as the cervix relaxes the placenta can be drawn out.

True retained placenta is caused by an adherent placenta (placenta accreta) and requires manual removal under high regional or general anaesthetic. Failure of placental separation due to uterine atony is rarely seen after Syntometrine.

Acute inversion of the uterus Causes heavy bleeding and immediate shock due to vagal stimulation. The fundus is felt in the vagina and is impalpable per abdomen. Replace immediately if possible, otherwise resuscitate and reduce hydrostatically with warm saline. Give antibiotics and Syntocinon to maintain contraction of uterus.

◆ Primary postpartum haemorrhage (PPH)

Primary PPH is defined as blood loss of more than 500 ml within 24 hours of delivery. The incidence is about 1%.

The *causes* are:
– atonic uterus
– retained placenta
– tear (vagina, cervix, uterus)
– DIC (rare)

Management
1. *Resuscitate* (i.v. infusion, crossmatch, consider plasma expanders while awaiting blood).
2. *Atonic uterus* is unusual now with routine Syntometrine. It can follow long labour, hydramnios, twins or abruption and is more likely with a history of previous PPH or APH in this pregnancy.

The uterus normally contracts firmly and compresses the vessels feeding the placental site. If the uterus is not firmly contracted, rub up a contraction (which will push out any clots) and repeat ergometrine (0.5 mg i.m. or i.v.) once. Call for help *early* (PPH still kills). A Syntocinon infusion (40 U in 500 ml saline) may be needed for a few hours to maintain contraction. If the uterus fails to contract, bimanual compression may be necessary as an emergency measure (one hand on the abdomen and a fist in the anterior fornix). Hemabate (PGF$_{2\alpha}$) given by injection directly into the myometrium can be life-saving.
3. *Retained placenta*: check that the placenta is complete. If any placenta is retained, the uterus will be unable to contract properly and manual removal under GA will be necessary.
4. If the uterus is empty and well contracted, the bleeding cannot be coming from the placental site and must be *traumatic*:
   – episiotomy
   – vaginal tear

- cervical tear
- uterine rupture

Full anaesthetic block (GA or spinal) is essential in every case to inspect the whole genital tract. Lacerations are sutured. If bleeding continues, uterine rupture is diagnosed and laparotomy performed (haemostatic suture or hysterectomy).

5. *DIC* occurs rarely – usually after placental abruption or severe pre-eclampsia, but also with sepsis – and can cause massive PPH. There is oozing from the venepuncture sites and the blood taken fails to clot in a plain sample container. FDPs are raised and fibrinogen will be low. It is treated with inotropic support, fresh frozen plasma, fresh whole blood and intensive medical support with care shared between obstetrician, anaesthetist and physician. Spontaneous improvement occurs after careful support.

   Note: In the home, call for paramedics and ambulance and alert on-call obstetric team. Never transfer a patient who is still bleeding. Repeat ergometrine, establish an i.v. infusion if possible, and maintain bimanual compression of the uterus until facilities are ready for exploration under GA.

6. PPH is particularly dangerous if the woman is already anaemic or has had a previous APH: 'APH harms, PPH kills'.

   Acute renal failure can occur and urine output must be monitored. If this is <30 ml/hour correct hypovolaemia, ideally with a CVP line, and give high-dose frusemide (e.g. *one* dose of 40 mg i.v. over 20 minutes) or mannitol (e.g. 50 ml of 25% mannitol over 20 minutes). If this fails to 'rescue' the tubules from necrosis, and oliguria persists, it is necessary to start a acute renal failure regime:
   - transfer to specialist unit (renal unit/ITU)
   - restrict fluids (500 ml + output of previous day)
   - high-carbohydrate low-protein diet (e.g. Hycal, 2500 kcal/day)
   - weigh daily (?fluid retention)
   - monitor U&E (potassium can rise – consider 100 ml of 50% dextrose with 20 U soluble insulin in emergency; ion-exchange resins or dialysis to remove)
   - monitor urine (volume, electrolytes)
   - 'renal' dose of dopamine i.v.
   - dialyse (fluid retention, urea above 50 mmol/l, potassium above 7 mmol/l)
   - await recovery, usually 1–2 weeks (keep up with polyuria)

7. Severe PPH can cause *primary necrosis* (rare) which can cause death or present as failure of lactation and subsequent amenorrhoea. Replacement cortisol and T4 are necessary (Simmonds' or Sheehan's syndrome).

◆ Maternal collapse and shock

The *possible mechanisms* of shock are:
- hypovolaemic (haemorrhage)
- endotoxic (septicaemia)
- cardiogenic (pulmonary embolus)

– anaphylactic (drugs, usually + bronchospasm)
– neurogenic (traction on viscera, uterine inversion)

In hypovolaemia decreased cardiac output causes catecholamine release with vasoconstriction in skin, kidneys and muscle (pallor, oliguria, tissue hypoxia and acidosis) which maintains the BP and perfusion pressure to the brain and heart.

Gram-negative septicaemia usually causes rigors and the endotoxins cause peripheral vasodilation (hence the skin is warm and red).

Obstetric shock is usually haemorrhagic:
– APH (placenta praevia, abruption)
– PPH (atonic uterus, retained placenta, trauma)
– uterine rupture

If septicaemia is a possibility, take blood culture and give high dose i.v. broad-spectrum antibiotics: DIC can occur.

Always suspect amniotic fluid embolism – after delivery or in late labour, grand multip with intact membranes, cyanosis, cough, sudden collapse. 50% are fatal.

Management
– summon adult resuscitation team
– oxygen, airway, output (wedge to l. lateral)
– i.v. fluids (preferably under CVP control)
– crossmatch
– oxygen
– diamorphine i.v. for pain and LVF
  consider antibiotics
– consider i.v. steroids (acute adrenal failure can occur secondary to shock)
– monitor urine output (?acute renal failure)

Amniotic fluid embolism
Very rare, but featured strongly in latest maternal death enquiries. Causes sudden shock and cyanosis at the height of a contraction. CVP is raised, CXR shows mottled opacities. It is often fatal. *Postmortem* reveals widespread DIC, diagnostic fetal squames (from amniotic fluid) in lungs.

Collapse after GA
Following GA consider:
– aspiration (CXR, blood gases show hypoxia)
– incompatible transfusion

In *incompatible transfusion*, the GA masks rigors, headache and loin pain. Haemolysis and anaphylactic shock occur. Stop infusion, resuscitate, send clotted blood (?Coombs positive, i.e. red cells coated with antibody) and collect urine (?oliguria, ?haemoglobinuria).

Uterine rupture
There are three clinical situations:
– *obstructed labour* (section should be performed for oblique lie or disproportion once there is failure to progress and long before the uterus ruptures)
– *ruptured scar* (the scar of a previous section can rupture in labour with sudden pain that continues between contractions and, usually,

signs of fetal distress – emergency section. Bleeding from the fibrous scar is often minimal)
- *PPH* (resuscitate and laparotomy, hysterectomy can be life-saving)

◆ Bonding

Bonding between mother and infant is essential for both physical growth and emotional development. Factors that promote attachment are:
- maternal feelings
- physical contact
- eye contact
- the baby's mimicry
- the baby's response to sound
- the baby's crying
- antenatal ultrasound is shown to enhance bonding

Note: Bonding with the father is also increasingly important especially as he is often present at delivery.

1. A natural anxiety about the child develops in most mothers during the early days and this promotes attachment.
   Maternal feelings vary and probably depend upon the quality of mothering the woman received as a child (the incidence of battering is increased in parents who were battered themselves).

2. *Close physical contact* is important for bonding and a mother will automatically touch and stroke the baby. She should be allowed to hold the infant at birth.
   Breastfeeding is the ideal way to promote physical contact and bonding. The baby can distinguish the smell of the mother's breast from 3 days.
   Unnecessary separation must be avoided. Mother and baby should share the same room 24 hours a day. There is evidence that the separation caused by SCBU increases the incidence of battering.

3. *Eye contact* is an important method of mother–infant communication. Mothers often feel particularly cut off from their child if he is blind or has his eyes covered during phototherapy.
   The child can see at birth, can follow moving objects, prefers patterned stimuli and focuses best at 30 cm. Hence breastfeeding provides the ideal position for eye contact. He can recognise his mother's face by 3 weeks.

4. *Mimicry of facial movements* such as mouth opening or tongue protrusion can sometimes start as early as the first week. The mother feels rewarded by these copied movements, and so in effect she is being encouraged by her baby to communicate.

5. The baby can hear from birth, and from a few days *responds particularly to his mother's voice*. Mothers talking to their baby invariably use high-pitched sounds. Analysis of film shows that the baby responds to his mother's voice by means of gestures and movements, and that a continuous interaction is occurring between them.

6. Sound spectrography confirms that cries of hunger and pain are different and *the baby uses crying to communicate demands for food, attention or physical contact* (cuddling). The baby thereby initiates further social interaction.

Bonding problems If the mother is reluctant to feed or handle her baby, or is preoccupied with her own symptoms rather than the care of the baby, these are warning signs that bonding is going to be a problem.

There may be an explanation such as a previous stillbirth or neonatal death, or it may be due to depression; the baby may be rather dull and unresponsive. Extra help from the staff can encourage normal bonding.

◆ Breast problems

- cracked nipples
- engorgement
- mastitis
- breast abscess
- poor supply of milk
- drugs
- galactocele

1. *Cracked nipples* means either a raw area or a fissure. Prevent by avoiding prolonged sucking (5–10 minutes each side is adequate). Make sure the infant is taking the whole nipple and areola well into the mouth (which decreases the shearing force on the skin of the nipple) and is not repeatedly releasing the nipple due to nasal obstruction (consider 1% ephedrine nose drops before feeds). Lanolin can be used to prevent excessive drying of the skin.

   If cracked nipple occurs, rest that breast and express milk, taking care with hygeine. Antiseptics such as chlorhexidine spray (Rotersept) are discouraged. Ointments such as Kamillosan may contain nut oils and may possibly increase later susceptibility to nut allergy. Cracked nipples usually heal in 48 hours when feeding can be gradually re-introduced. If persistent, consider thrush. Nipple shields may help.

2. *Breast engorgement* is common on days 3–4 (as oestrogen levels fall, prolactin stimulates milk secretion). It is less likely to occur if the nipples are washed regularly in later pregnancy, because colostrum is secreted from 28 weeks and the ducts can get blocked. Both breasts become distended, hard, tender and painful and the woman is febrile.

   Express milk (the electric pump is less painful than manual expression), give analgesia, support with firm bra and avoid nipple stimulation. If severe, and breastfeeding is not desired, lactation can be suppressed with bromocriptine, 2.5 mg b.d. for 10 days.

3. *Mastitis*. Breast pain, fever, and a tender, red, wedge-shaped area on the breast. It usually follows a cracked nipple, and the baby may have an infected umbilicus. The organism is almost always *Staph. aureus* (swabs and milk can be sent for culture).

   Treat with immediate flucloxacillin 500 mg q.d.s. and analgesia. Breastfeeding can continue unless too painful. Isolate mother and infant.

4. *Breast abscess*. Mastitis worsens with brawny oedema and axillary lymphadenopathy. Stop breastfeeding and suppress lactation with bromocriptine 2.5 mg b.d. Prompt surgical drainage via a radial incision is necessary, and a drainage tube is inserted.

Swab pus and continue flucloxacillin until the results of culture are known.

5. *Poor milk supply*. The stimuli for secretion of milk are:
   - nipple stimulation
   - breast emptying

   High fluid intake is necessary. Feed on demand to increase suckling, and express milk at the end of each feed. Only if the baby is thirsty give 5% dextrose or water between feeds. Test-weighing before and after each feed for 24 hours usually makes the mother anxious but proves whether or not the baby is getting sufficient milk (approximately 150 ml/kg/day). If insufficient breast milk is available, complementary bottle feeds can be given after each breastfeed to make up the amount.

6. *Drugs*. Most drugs are only excreted in very small quantities in breastmilk. It is safe to continue breastfeeding if the mother is on heparin or warfarin, phenytoin, anti-inflammatories, bronchodilator inhalers, hypotensives, digoxin, steroids and most antibiotics (although drugs should obviously be avoided if possible). Metronidazole is safe but gives the milk a bitter taste. Paracetamol is safe.

   If the mother is on carbimazole, monitor the baby's thyroxine. Lithium, ^{131}I and cytotoxics are contraindications to breastfeeding. Barbiturates, benzodiazepines, ephedrine, opiates and stimulant laxatives can all harm the baby and should be avoided. Breastfeeding is safe after rubella vaccination and with low-dose oestrogen pills (which do not suppress lactation).

7. *Galactocele*. A non-tender retention cyst of milk that usually needs excision (to exclude carcinoma).

◆ Puerperal fever

Epidemic childbed fever (puerperal sepsis) was largely due to infection with haemolytic streptococci and used to be almost as feared as labour itself. Semmelweiss observed in 1861 that the disease could be passed by the unwashed hands of doctors from case to case, and wrote: 'God only knows how many women I have prematurely brought down into the grave'.

Temperatures above 38°C within 14 days of delivery were notifiable until the early 1980s: a midwife is still obliged to refer the patient to a doctor if the temperature is above 37.5°C for more than 3 days. Even maternity units opened in the late 1980s had puerperal sepsis wards. Infection remains a real hazard. *Consider*:
- genital tract infection
- UTI
- breasts (engorgement, mastitis)
- episiotomy site
- superficial phlebitis (treat with aspirin)
- DVT
- chest infection (usually post-GA in a smoker)
- unrelated (influenza, tonsillitis)

Examine breasts, chest, abdomen, perineum and legs and take:
- HVS
- MSU
- blood cultures (if diagnosis uncertain)
- (throat swab)

The raw placental site is effectively an open wound and is predisposed to infection. *Puerperal sepsis* causes fever (usually within 24 hours of delivery) with foul lochia, and the uterus may be tender. The usual organisms are:
- streptococci
- coliforms
- anaerobes

Take an HVS (rigors suggest septicaemia – take blood cultures) and start antibiotics (e.g. Augmentin or cefuroxime and metronidazole).

Low abdominal pain and tenderness suggest pelvic peritonitis that may go on to form a pelvic abscess requiring surgical drainage.

◆ Deep vein thrombosis (DVT)

The incidence of venous thrombosis is increased at least ×5 in pregnancy, and fatal thromboembolism remains the most common cause of maternal death. The incidence is particularly high in women who have had a prolonged period of antenatal bedrest and who are then delivered by section. *The increased incidence of thrombosis in pregnancy is due to:*
- increased fibrinogen and Factors V, VIII, X
- decreased plasminogen activity (clots not lysed)
- venous stasis in legs (pressure from the uterus)

Diagnosis   The clinical diagnosis of DVT is notoriously unreliable. Thrombosis is silent in 50% of cases and *the signs* can occur without thrombosis:
- calf pain
- calf tenderness, Homans' sign
- femoral pain and tenderness
- oedema, dilated veins
- swelling (increased circumference)
- warmth of leg
- low-grade fever

Note: Femoral pain and tenderness are the most reliable signs.

Features suggestive of *pulmonary embolus* are dyspnoea (if small and scattered), pleuritic pain and haemoptysis (if moderate) or shock (if massive). Lung scan within 24 hours may show an area of decreased perfusion but pulmonary angiography is necessary for definitive diagnosis. Treatment is with heparin (or streptokinase and embolectomy if massive and postnatal).

If the *diagnosis* of DVT is in doubt it is justifiable to wait for 24–48 hours, because the incidence of pulmonary embolus is low in DVT below the knee, and if due to other causes the symptoms may settle. Pelvic DVT requires prompt and aggressive management.

If the thrombosis seems to be extending then a *venogram* is indicated to confirm the diagnosis. Confirmation is important before subjecting the woman to prolonged anticoagulation.

Ultrasound techniques are less accurate, especially in pregnancy when the gravid uterus retards flow in the femoral veins.

Injecting *labelled fibrinogen* to identify a thrombus is contraindicated in pregnancy and during breastfeeding.

Treatment

Use full-length elastic stocking (to improve venous flow), elevation of the leg, analgesia and *anticoagulation*.

Intravenous *heparin* by infusion pump (5000 U stat then 10 000–15 000 U 6-hourly) prevents extension of the clot. This is continued for 48–72 hours, then warfarin is continued for at least 3 months. In adult medicine generally there is a move toward outpatient management of DVT with subcutaneous low molecular weight heparins. This remains unproven in the obstetric case – inpatient assessment is always wise, and traditional i.v. heparin, at least to begin with, is probably preferable.

Changing from heparin to warfarin: give a loading dose of warfarin (usually 10 mg daily for 2 days) on the morning of day 2 of heparin treatment. Stop heparin on the evening of day 3 (so it does not interfere with the APTT test) and measure the APTT on the morning of day 4. According to the results, the haematology lab will advise on the correct dose of warfarin (usually 2–5 mg) to be given on the evening of day 4. Daily tests can be performed to find the correct maintenance dose of warfarin.

Warfarin therapy is *monitored* by APTT (aim for 2.0–2.5 times longer than normal). Postnatal mothers may choose to remain on heparin as this avoids repeated hospital blood-test monitoring. Check local guidelines.

Note: Warfarin does not increase blood loss from a well-contracted uterus. Breastfeeding is perfectly safe during heparin or warfarin therapy, as only minute quantities cross into the milk.

Antenatally: warfarin crosses the placenta, heparin does not.

Prophylactic anticoagulation

During pregnancy prophylactic anticoagulation is indicated if there is a past history of proven DVT.

Self-administered subcutaneous heparin, 5000 U b.d. or t.d.s, or low molecular weight heparins can be used (e.g. Clexane 20–40 mg daily) because heparin does not cross the placenta. It decreases the incidence of recurrent thrombosis by inhibiting activated Factor X (it has no effect on APTT).

It is stopped as soon as labour starts (it has a short half-life of about 6 hours), then recommenced about 6 hours later and continued for 2 weeks.

If a woman develops a *DVT in pregnancy* it should be confirmed by venogram if possible (the fetus can be protected by a lead shield) and i.v. heparin infusion is given in the usual way, before changing to subcutaneous heparin.

Warfarin can be used in pregnancy – e.g. for women with prosthetic heart valves, for whom heparins are unsuitable. During the first 12 weeks it can be teratogenic (nasal hypoplasia and nail changes).

Safest use is between 12 and 37 weeks, but fetal intracranial haemorrhages are still a risk. In heart valve patients the benefits outweigh the risks but should be carefully discussed.

Prolonged (> 12 weeks) heparin use can lead to radiological evidence of osteoporosis, increasingly a risk if prolonged breastfeeding as well: with past history of DVT, therefore, most advise beginning prophylaxis from 36 weeks gestation to 6 weeks postpartum rather than treatment right through pregnancy.

Proven previous PE may justify commencement of warfarin or early heparin. Warfarin should be stopped at 37 weeks and changed to heparin because warfarin crosses the placenta (and anticoagulates the fetus, with an increased risk of large intracranial haemorrhage during delivery).

If premature labour occurs, clotting factors should be replenished with fresh frozen plasma.

The baby should receive vitamin K if warfarin used.

◆ Secondary PPH

1. Defined as *bleeding after 24 hours and up to 6 weeks after delivery*. It usually occurs around days 10–14. The lochia should gradually be getting lighter by this time and any recurrence of bleeding is abnormal.
2. The *cause* is usually a retained piece of placenta ± infection.
3. *Features*: usually the lochia remain heavy, the uterus fails to involute and the cervix is open. With infection there is offensive lochia and fever.
4. *Treatment*: with moderate loss and minimal suspicion of retained products it is common to give *ergometrine* 0.5 mg t.d.s. orally for 2 days (although there is little proven benefit) and *antibiotics* (e.g. Augmentin and metronidazole). Ultrasound scan can sometimes demonstrate retained products but can confuse blood and products – decision for surgery therefore remains a clinical one.

   If loss is heavy, *surgical evacuation* of retained products of conception (ERPC) is necessary. Occasionally, secondary PPH can be torrential and if the woman has sudden fresh bleeding (e.g. heavier than a period) she should be re-admitted immediately.
5. Early commencement of the POP often causes some breakthrough bleeding (spotting). If troublesome, stop the pill for a month and advise the sheath meantime.

◆ Puerperal depression

Mild postnatal 'depression' affects over 50%. These 'third day blues' consist of exhaustion, feeling weepy, mood swings, irritability, poor concentration and headaches. They last from a few hours to 7–10 days. Rising prolactin levels or falling endorphin levels are suggested causes but no causal hormonal change has been identified. About 10% go on to true depression.

◆ Puerperal psychosis

Tearfulness around days 3–4 is normal. Poor sleeping, rejecting the baby, distractability, multiple symptomatology or bizarre behaviour may signal impending psychosis.

The incidence of acute psychosis is increased for the 8 weeks following delivery and is about 1 in 1000. It tends to recur. Most psychiatric hospitals have mother-and-baby units for puerperal psychosis.

The *main features of psychosis* are:

1. Changes in behaviour, mood or conversation (e.g. fragmented speech or illogical associations).
2. Feeling emotionally distant (depersonalisation) or cut off from reality (derealisation).
3. *Thought control* – feeling that thoughts are being put into one's mind or removed from one's mind or are known to others.
4. Feelings of passivity – feeling that one is being controlled by some external person or thing.
5. *Delusions* – illogical and unshakeable beliefs, e.g. 'that television programme contains secret instructions'.
6. *Auditory hallucinations* – voices, usually discussing the person, e.g. 'she is disgusting; she is under my control'.

If suspected, an urgent psychiatric assessment is necessary. There is some evidence that progesterone (suppositories or i.m.) late in the third trimester and postnatally reduces the recurrence of postnatal depression (Dalton's work was on i.m. progesterones initially; later on rectal use). Worth a try as there is no risk.

◆ The immediate postnatal period

Check the following:
– clinical: temp, pulse, BP, fundus and lochia, sutures, breasts, passed urine, feeding technique (avoid problems), analgesia, bowels, legs (DVT)
– Hb
– rubella status – check vaccination not needed
– Rhesus – is anti-D needed? (within 72 hours max)
– baby check ± paediatrician (or GP) to check baby

Tachycardia suggests anaemia or infection. Following PET the BP is usually normal and proteinuria resolved by 48 hours. If not, arrange follow-up and possibly renal function tests.

Contractions continue, especially on breastfeeding (after-pains) and may require analgesia. *Perineal bruising* can be painful and analgesia, ice or ultrasound can help. A dry sterile vulval pad is changed regularly to prevent infection. *Early ambulation* is encouraged to prevent DVT.

The fundus involutes rapidly:
day 1 – 24 weeks size (umbilicus)
day 5 – 16 weeks size
day 10 – impalpable

Slow involution should be noted (but ignored if lochia and temperature are normal). A persistent bulky uterus may be due to retained products (visible on scan) and requires evacuation.

Anaemia: if Hb is checked too soon, it is of little value, but circumstances usually dictate timing. If concerned, recheck after day 5. If Hb is below 10 g/dl continue oral iron for 3 months. Usually need to transfuse if symptomatic or Hb less than 8 g/dl.

If the mother is *Rhesus-negative (with no antibodies)* and the baby is Rhesus-positive, then anti-D (usually 500 IU) is given i.m. within 72 hours of delivery.

If the woman has no *rubella antibodies* she should be immunised, with strict contraception (e.g. Depo-Provera) for 3 months. Breast-feeding is safe.

Note the *mental state*.

Discuss *contraception*, which is still necessary during breastfeeding. The POP is used instead of the combined pill if breastfeeding (oestrogens suppress lactation) and can be started on discharge. The IUD and the diaphragm need to be refitted at 6 weeks, after complete involution of the uterus.

Sterilisation is normally delayed 3–4 months (by then tubes less vascular and any abnormalities of the infant are apparent: laparoscopic procedure then much safer than postpartum tubal ligation).

Discuss any problems. The *district midwife* may visit the home every day for the first 10 days to: check temperature, fundus, perineum and bowels, to give advice on feeding, to ensure cord care; and to perform the Guthrie test. She can continue visits to day 28 if she feels it necessary.

The *health visitor* visits after day 11 to discuss future immunisations and the role of the baby clinic, and she is responsible for future developmental assessments.

◆ The 6-week postnatal examination

The GP should visit mother and baby at least once within 7 days of delivery. The routine postnatal examination of the mother at 6 weeks has developed the reputation for being a largely unnecessary ritual. In fact, most women like to attend and it serves several useful functions.

– query symptoms (stress incontinence, dyspareunia)
– discuss anxieties
– follow-up of complications
– contraception and smear
– VE (if symptomatic)
– 6-week infant screening
– assess mother–infant bonding
– complete paperwork and register the child in the practice
– ? arrange discussion with hospital if complicated delivery

Notes   1. Pelvic floor exercises will overcome minor postpartum stress incontinence and should be explained by the doctor or physiotherapist.

Dyspareunia after episiotomy repair almost always settles without the need for surgery. If real problems refer early – marital strain is worsened by sexual difficulty. Primary wound breakdown is best managed expectantly – re-suturing is often unsuccessful (infection) and healing by secondary intention is good.

Always ask specifically about urinary and faecal/flatal continence or soiling. 50% of women have symptoms for more than 6 months and most do not mention them. Refer early to urogynaecology or for colorectal surgical opinion.

179

2. *Specific anxieties* can be fully discussed, e.g. concerning the need for future sections, or following a perinatal death or fetal abnormality – the couple may need referral for genetic counselling.

3. *Specific antenatal complications* may need follow-up:
   - hypertension
   - anaemia
   - recurrent UTIs (consider IVU or renal USS after 12 weeks)
   - gestational glucose intolerance (arrange postnatal GTT)

4. *Contraception* will already have been discussed and a majority of women will be on the pill. However, the diaphragm and IUD are not refitted until 6 weeks. Sterilisation may be requested. A *smear* may be due or the date of the next smear can be arranged.

5. *VE* is unnecessary if the woman is asymptomatic following a normal delivery. Erosion and retroversion are very common postpartum and can be ignored.

6. *The 6-week assessment of the infant* normally takes 2–3 minutes: it is a useful time to discuss minor problems (e.g. skin blemishes), exclude abnormalities and reassure the mother that the baby is normal. (See also Chapter 5.)
   a) Ask about:
      - birth (gestation, weight, delivery)
      - sucking and feeding
      - excessive sleeping or crying
      - smiling (average 4–6 weeks)

      Note: Smiling in response to social overtures (i.e. when talked to) is a reassuring sign of normality.
   b) Note general alertness (an important sign).
   c) Examine mouth (thrush), eyes (squint, nystagmus), heart (murmur) and umbilicus (infection).
   d) Ventral suspension on one hand (the baby should lift its head momentarily and extend the legs) and note any dermal sinus. Pull to sitting (head-lag should no longer be complete). Test for ankle clonus. Examine the hips (see section on CDH in Chapter 5).
   e) Growth chart. Plot weight and head circumference for birth and 6 weeks – they should both be on the same centile. If the head is abnormally large examine fontanelles and sutures and consider referral for assessment (and possible CT scan and possible shunt).

      There is wide normal variation in development and even definitely abnormal signs may disappear. Features that IN COMBINATION may suggest some degree of mental subnormality or cerebral palsy, and indicate the need for increased developmental surveillance are:
      - prematurity or birth asphyxia
      - decreased alertness, excessive sleeping
      - poor sucking, irritability
      - late smiling
      - one limb feels stiff, hand kept closed
      - movements decreased or asymmetrical
      - excessive head-lag, brisk knee jerks, ankle clonus

7. Assessment of maternal attitude to the baby is important. Poor bonding can lead to emotional deprivation, which causes failure to thrive.
8. Postnatal visits by GPs attract a fee, and the full postnatal examination at around 6 weeks attracts a further, higher fee.

When the parents register the birth, the registrar gives them a card which they should bring to register their child with the general practitioner.

◆ Alternative methods of childbirth

The rationale for the active management of labour is that it keeps mother and baby as safe as possible. 50 years ago the maternal mortality rate was 5 per 1000 and about 1 in 20 babies died. It is now assumed that women are willing to tolerate the restrictions of a hospital delivery in the knowledge that safety is assured, as far as is possible.

However, current obstetric practice is being increasingly questioned. Some women complain that having a baby involves being 'processed' by the medical system, that much of the routine management is unnecessary or even harmful and spoils the enjoyment of childbirth. The medical intervention necessary for a minority of complicated labours has spilled over onto the majority of normal deliveries.

A movement for non-intervention or 'active birth' is growing. Its aims are to support the right of women to make informed decisions about how they want to give birth, and to encourage the professionals to provide information, help and support in such a way as to further that aim.

In the quest for safety, obstetrics has evolved to become very different from the methods of childbirth seen in primitive cultures. In remote tribes in New Guinea and South Africa, women squat outdoors to deliver a baby. They are supported, massaged and comforted by other women. The baby is not touched until completely out of the vagina, the cord is cut but not tied, and the mother assumes immediate responsibility for the child.

The perinatal mortality in such primitive communities is around 50 per 1000. It is sometimes argued that any deviation away from our current methods might once more increase the dangers. There is no evidence for this in low-risk women.

However, units such as that of Michel Odent in France have demonstrated that alternative methods of management *can* be perfectly safe. In that particular unit the emphasis is on allowing the woman freedom to do as she feels. Labour is never induced or augmented, the woman can be mobile throughout labour and she can choose her own position for delivery (usually squatting). No drugs or epidurals are used (a warm bath is recommended for severe pain and also appears to help cervical dilatation). Forceps are not used. Vacuum extraction is occasionally used (5%). There is only a 6% episiotomy rate and a 6% caesarean rate. The techniques of Leboyer (intended to minimise the trauma of delivery for the baby) are also used: quietness, dim lighting, delivery into water, and delayed cutting of the cord. The perinatal mortality rate in 1980 was only 7 per 1000.

181

Water for pain relief
and birth   Michel Odent installed a birthing pool in his French unit in 1976. In 1992, a House of Commons committee recommended that all hospitals should allow women the option of a birthing pool. It offers:
- freedom of movement and position (weightlessness)
- peace, private space, warmth, calming effect
- enhanced relaxation – better endorphin production and possibly increased oxytocin production

It is suitable for:
- normal pregnancy > 37 weeks
- expectation of normal outcome
- established labour (> 4 cm)

Caution: If SROM, delivery should be within 24 hours. Do CTG beforehand

Care in the pool   - $\frac{1}{2}$-hourly observations – temperature, pulse, BP
- water temperature should be within the mother's comfort range; 36–37°C. if the mother becomes hyperthermic and tachycardic the baby will react to these changes in a similar fashion. Keep ambient room temperature lower
- keep water level just below her breasts
- listen to the FH every 15 minutes for 1 minute in the first stage (underwater sonicaid is ideal)
- use partogram as normal
- allow plenty of oral fluids to avoid dehydration
- glucose sweets avoid ketosis
- tepid sponging reduces overheating
- Entonox is useful

Delivery   (Some women will leave the pool to deliver.)
- auscultate the FH after every contraction for 1 minute in the second stage
- the head crowns slowly and protecting the perineum is usually not necessary
- tangled cord releases easily in water
- avoid stimulating the baby under water – don't touch
- lift baby immediately to the surface
- keep baby warm – will breathe when air is reached
- never cut/clamp the cord while the baby is under water

Third stage   - PPH remains a risk – active or physiological management should be discussed as usual
- perineal suturing, if required, is delayed for about an hour as the tissues are waterlogged and difficult to handle

◆ 'Routine' obstetric practices – what is right?

All aspects of care are being increasingly questioned. Is the supine position, recommended for the past 300 years (and certainly easier for vaginal examination) really the best during labour? Being mobile (so that gravity helps to dilate the cervix) and changing position frequently (with less obstruction to the IVC) would seem sensible, and some research suggests that labour is then shorter and less painful. The advent of radiotelemetry will make this possible even if fetal monitoring is necessary.

Is pethidine overused? Since 1853, when John Snow used chloroform for the delivery of Queen Victoria's eighth child, Prince Leopold, methods of pain relief in labour have received great emphasis.

Both pethidine and epidural anaesthesia restrict mobility and there are various drug-free methods of pain control that can be very effective, including focused concentration, relaxation techniques, emotional support, position changes, breath control, massage, yoga, meditation, acupressure, acupuncture and hypnosis.

It is well known that good antenatal education and familiarity with surroundings and birth attendants help to prevent the ignorance–fear–tension–pain cycle. Should we be doing more?

Do the benefits of early amniotomy and fetal monitoring in an otherwise normal labour really outweigh the disadvantages of immobility and the risk of infection?

Is it really vital that all women in labour must starve and have i.v. dextrose for ketonuria?

Is the lithotomy position with commanded pushing really the best for delivery? Given the choice, many women prefer to squat, and there is some evidence that in this position the contractions are more effective and oxygenation of the fetus is improved.

Does an episiotomy really heal better than a larger tear and cause less subsequent dyspareunia? The evidence begins to suggest that it does not.

Is a sterile field important for delivery? Would the mother touching the baby as it is born really cause infection?

Is Syntometrine essential for *every* woman? Placenta separation is also accelerated by allowing the placental end of the cord to drain blood and by immediate maternal suckling. Some people feel that Syntometrine increases the chances of retained membranes and delayed involution.

Should the mucus extractor be used routinely? Most babies sneeze up excess mucus and the extractor can sometimes delay the onset of respiration if used too vigorously.

Women should ideally be able to make informed decisions about how they want to have their own baby. Some women feel reassured by a fully equipped labour ward. Others want a minimum of interference (a State Registered Midwife must attend the delivery under the 1951 Midwives Act).

Birth plans   Sheila Kitzinger promoted the idea of a 'birth plan'. Early in pregnancy (or even in the preconception clinic) the woman should have the opportunity to learn about the various options and to consider what would be most suitable for her.

The following issues are important:
- where she wants to have the baby
- what sort of pain relief she would prefer
- how much intervention or supervision she would wish
- what the routine procedures are at the local maternity hospital

- what does she feel about early amniotomy and fetal monitoring
- will she be allowed to move around in labour and choose her delivery position?
- whether she wants an episiotomy
- whether she will be separated from the baby after delivery
- what will happen if complications arise and a caesarean section is necessary or the baby has to be cared for on the SCBU?
- how long would she like to stay in hospital?
- can her partner stay?

Of course, not all women would be interested in thinking ahead in such detail, but a birth plan would help midwives to provide the personalised service that most already aim to achieve.

The ideal would be a system of care (including advanced medical technology where necessary) that is flexible enough to allow each woman to choose her own style of childbirth; that adapts to the woman's needs even as labour progresses, and that does not intrude on a couple's intimate experience of childbirth.

◆ References

Recent reports on Maternity Services

1. RCOG, RCM and RCGP. Maternity Care in the New NHS. 1992.
2. Cumberledge Report. Changing Childbirth: Report of the Expert Maternity Group. HMSO; 1993.
3. DOH. The Patient's Charter and Maternity Services. 1994.
4. RCOG. Organisational Standards for Maternity Services. 1995.
5. Reports on Confidential Enquiries into Maternal Deaths. HMSO. (Latest report, 'Why Mothers Die' covers 1994–96.)
6. RCOG and RCM Towards Safer Chidbirth – Minimum Standards of care on Labour Wards. 1999.
7. Confidential Enquiries into Stillbirths and Deaths in Infancy, (CESDI). Maternal and Child health consortium: June 2000. (The latest is 7th annual report, which includes 1998 statistics and focus group work on breech presentation in labour, and obstetric anaesthesia.)
8. RCM, RCOG and RCPCH. Reconfiguring maternity services, July 2000.

Other publications of interest to GPs

1. RCOG. Intimate Examinations: Working Party report. 1997.
2. RCPCH. Resuscitation of Babies at Birth.
3. GMC Seeking Patients' Consent: the Ethical Considerations. (Also practical advice by Defence Organisations.)
4. GMC Confidentiality: Guidance from GMC.
5. GMC. Serious Communicable Diseases.

The latest clinical guidelines may be found on the RCOG website: http:// www.rcog.org.uk

5. The neonate

◆ The fetal circulation

There are two *shunts* which allow blood to bypass the lungs:
- the foramen ovale
- the patent ductus

1. Oxygenated blood via the umbilical vein and IVC enters the right atrium and passes through the *foramen ovale* to the left side of the heart to supply the head and neck.
2. Blood returning from the head and neck in the SVC enters the right atrium from above and tends to flow into the right ventricle and pulmonary artery and then through the *patent ductus* to the lower aorta, the rest of the body and umbilical arteries back to the placenta.

At birth the lungs expand, pulmonary vascular resistance falls and blood is sucked from the right side of the heart and returned to the left atrium, therefore closing the foramen ovale. The PO_2 then rises and causes spasm of the ductus (prostaglandin-mediated) and umbilical vessels. (Hence in RDS with a low PO_2 there is often a persistent ductus murmur.) The ductus can be kept patent by giving prostaglandin E_2 (e.g. in total transposition prior to surgery).

◆ Neonatal resuscitation

7% of infants require intubation at birth, but only 50% of these can be predicted by known risk factors (twins, diabetes, Rhesus disease, premature labour, fetal distress, breech, difficult forceps, section). This implies that intrapartum fetal monitoring should be available for all deliveries. Severe asphyxia causes cerebral palsy but the relationship between the need for resuscitation and later learning difficulties or cerebral palsy is unknown.

The *Apgar score* (Table 7) is routinely assessed at 1, 5 and 10 minutes and is a numerical assessment of the baby's condition at birth.

Table 7 Assessing condition at birth

	0	1	2
Pulse	Absent	Below 100	Above 100
Respiration	Absent	Irregular	Crying
Colour	Pale or blue	Pink + blue extremities	Pink
Tone	Limp	Slight flexion	Active
Grimace	None	Grimaces	Cries

185

It is not particularly helpful in predicting which babies require resuscitation because this decision is only based on respiration and pulse rate and needs to be made within that first 60 seconds. The other features scored are colour, tone and grimace response to pharyngeal stimulation. Since all babies have some peripheral cyanosis, the maximum score is 9 at birth.

Resuscitation
procedure

1. Prior to delivery, switch on the radiant heater on the resuscitaire. Check the oxygen supply, the suction and the laryngoscope.
2. Clear the airway. Aspirate the pharynx with a suction catheter and give facial oxygen while the tongue is blue. For most babies it is sufficient to wipe the lips and nose with a piece of gauze.
3. Keep the baby warm by drying the infant and placing under the radiant heater.
4. Assess colour, heart rate and respiration. The baby will fall into one of the three following groups:
   - pink, regular respirations, heart rate > 100 – healthy baby, keep warm and give to mother
   - blue, inadequate respirations, heart rate > 100 – clear airway, if no response, further resuscitation is required
   - blue or white, apnoeic, heart rate < 100 – needs prompt resuscitation
5. If there is no breathing by 30 seconds, use a self-inflating bag and a close-fitting mask to inflate the lungs a few times to start off spontaneous breathing.
6. If not breathing by 60 seconds, intubate.
7. If heart rate falls below 100 at any time, this signifies hypoxia. External cardiac massage is required if the rate falls below 60 (rate 120, ratio 3:1). Oxygenation by mask is often sufficient to restore the pulse, otherwise intubation is indicated.
8. After intubation suck out secretions with a fine catheter. Low-pressure IPPV (<30 cm H_2O) is used to induce reflex inspiratory movements and success is judged by a return of a normal pulse rate within 15–30 seconds.

   If this does not occur, continue external cardiac massage until the heart rate is > 100, check breath sounds (unilateral if tube passed down into the right main bronchus), check the connections, consider naloxone (0.01 mg/kg) if the mother had pethidine and order a chest X-ray (diaphragmatic hernia, pulmonary hypoplasia). Stop ventilating every 3 minutes to see if spontaneous breathing will continue.
9. Empty the stomach to prevent later aspiration.
10. If the baby has a bradycardia despite adequate ventilation check the pH and give colloid if acidotic.

Outcome

Most babies can go to the routine postnatal ward after successful resuscitation. If it was prolonged they are observed on SCBU for several hours first. Reassure the parents.

If unsuccessful, explain to the parents, and encourage them to hold the dead infant. If staff have the courage and kindness to be with the parents and help them say goodbye to their child it greatly helps their later bereavement. Inform their GP.

The outcome for a baby with no spontaneous cardiac output 15 minutes after the onset of cardiac arrest is likely to be very poor.

◆ Birth trauma

Intracranial haemorrhage

Torn falx due to large head or precipitate or breech delivery. The baby may either present with fits, irritability and a high-pitched cry, or can be lethargic, not feeding and having apnoeic attacks. The baby is observed on SCBU, phenobarbitone or phenytoin is used to control fits, blood sugar and calcium are measured, and an LP performed to exclude meningitis.

Intraventricular haemorrhage

A real-time ultrasound probe over the anterior fontanelle gives good views of the ventricular system. Research studies show that up to 40% of babies born before 33 weeks gestation suffer intraventricular haemorrhage in the first 3 days. They are usually small and sub-ependymal. Larger haemorrhages may be suspected clinically from apnoea, acidosis, hypotension or bulging fontanelle and can be confirmed by ultrasound. If the haemorrhage extends into the ventricles it can block CSF flow and cause ventricular dilation which, if severe, may need a shunt procedure.

Cephalhaematoma

Usually noticed at day 3. It is subperiosteal and limited by sutures (unlike caput). Rarely it can be large and require transfusion (the absorbed blood can worsen jaundice). Even if there is an associated depressed fracture there is usually no brain damage but it can leave a hard swelling that takes months to resolve.

Facial palsy

Not only due to forceps. Sometimes there is an area of subcutaneous fat necrosis on the face which resembles an abscess. It resolves in 2–3 weeks and meanwhile the exposed cornea must be protected with hypromellose drops.

Sternomastoid tumour

A lump (haematoma then fibroma) that develops in the lower part of the sternomastoid. It is associated with sternomastoid shortening and turns the head to the contralateral side. It appears around day 7 and is gone within 1 year. The mother can be taught passive movements to decrease the chance of later torticollis, which otherwise develops in about 10% around the age of 5 years.

Shoulder injuries

Lack of spontaneous or reflex movement in one arm. X-ray to exclude fractured clavicle (no treatment) or fractured humerus which is treated by splinting the arm to the chest with a crêpe bandage.

Brachial plexus injury is usually C5, C6 causing a 'waiter's tip' posture (Erb's palsy). Passive movements and sometimes splints are used to prevent contractures.

The degree of damage is always unknown but the prognosis is usually poor if signs persist after 6 months.

◆ Ambiguous genitalia

When a baby is born the parents usually ask two questions – 'Is it normal?' 'Is it a boy or a girl?'. The genitalia may look female but with labial fusion and an enlarged clitoris, or they may look male with hypospadias and undescended testes. THE CARDINAL RULE: never hazard a guess to placate the parents. Chromosomal analysis and other investigations to establish the sex take up to 1 week but the final decision on sex of rearing may not be possible for months. It is important to defer registration of the birth but not advisable to choose a name which is suitable for either sex.

There are three common possibilities:

1. *XX with congenital adrenal hyperplasia (CAH).* This is the commonest cause. All babies with ambiguous genitalia must have electrolytes monitored in case they have salt-losing CAH. It presents around day 3–7 as maternal steroid levels fall. A raised serum 17-hydroxyprogesterone confirms the diagnosis. Lifelong treatment with cortisone and mineralocorticoid is necessary; reproduction is possible.

2. *XY with partial masculinisation* due to an enzyme defect in the synthetic pathway of testosterone (one form is also salt-losing). The internal organs are male (complete or incomplete), and the external appearance varies from hypospadias to a little 'girl' with no vagina and inguinal lumps (testes) or herniae.

   The sex chosen depends on the internal anatomy (ultrasound scans and urethro-vaginagram) and on the anatomy of the external genitalia, and must be discussed with the surgeon.

   Generally, it is easier to construct a vagina than a penis, in which case the testes are excised and oestrogen given at puberty.

3. *Abnormal gonads* (very rare). This may be true *hermaphroditism* (XX and XY) with one testicle and one ovary (or bilateral ovotestes) or due to *mosaicism* (XX/XY). Internal organs are mixed. Again the anatomy of the external genitalia is usually the deciding factor.

◆ Congenital abnormalities

- spina bifida
- congenital dislocation of the hip
- hydrocephalus
- microcephaly
- cleft lip or palate
- congenital heart disease
- oesophageal atresia
- anorectal anomalies
- talipes

Spina bifida   Spina bifida occulta occurs in 10% of adult spines. In spina bifida cystica the dorsal laminae are absent and a dysplastic spinal cord protrudes through, producing a bulge on the back – a *myelomeningocele*. (In 5% the underlying cord is normal and the bulge is just a meningocele, which can be simply repaired.) The *problems* are:

1. 80% develop *hydrocephalus* due to an associated Arnold-Chiari malformation (compressing the aqueduct). It can be successfully treated by a shunt and 65% of shunted children have a normal IQ.
2. *Other associated congenital abnormalities* (cardiac, renal, gut).
3. *Paralysis*. With thoracic lesions the legs do not move and the child will never walk. With lumbar lesions the psoas muscles may be functioning and by transferring the psoas to extend the hip the child may walk with full-length calipers. With low lumbar lesions transfer to the tibialis anterior may enable walking with short calipers.
4. *Sensory loss* predisposes to pressure sores which may require skin grafts.
5. The *sacral nerves are always damaged*, with urinary retention, overflow, recurrent UTIs and hydronephrosis. An ileal conduit may be considered later in a girl. A patulous anus means there will be faecal incontinence.

If the child survives he will need repeated hospitalisation and probably several operations. Early repair of the back protects the neural plate from further damage but does not improve the neurological deficit.

The *indications for active treatment* have changed over the years. The Holter valve was introduced in 1958 and revolutionised the treatment of spina bifida. Unselective treatment of all children, however, resulted in severe multisystem handicap for survivors. Babies with an adverse prognosis can be selected on day 1 and should not receive active treatment. The criteria (often called the *Lorber criteria*) are:

– thoraco-lumbar lesions
– severe paraplegia
– gross head enlargement
– kyphosis or scoliosis
– other severe congenital defects or birth injuries

In spina bifida, hydrocephalus and anencephaly there is a 1 in 20 chance of a second affected child, 1 in 10 of a third. Screening for maternal serum AFP has reduced the incidence of neural tube defects.

Congenital dislocation of the hip

One in 200 births. Commoner in girls and after breech deliveries. There is often a family history.

Diagnosis

First the hips are abducted gently through 80°. If a hip is already dislocated there is resistance to abduction, then it reduces with a jolt (Ortolani's test). Next, Barlow's test is performed to re-dislocate it (performed on one hip at a time): with the hip flexed and slightly adducted, two movements are performed simultaneously, holding the greater trochanter between finger and thumb:

– push gently down towards the bed and up towards the baby's head
– internally rotate the hand 25°

The dislocated hip feels as if it is 'moving into gear'. 10% of hips click, but if there is no abnormal movement it is ignored.

Management CDH is treated with a Von Rosen splint. This is a malleable, padded, H-shaped frame which the baby wears *under* nappies from the second day. It is checked daily at first to prevent pressure points by padding and to check abduction is being held, then fortnightly to adjust the abduction as the baby grows (excess can cause avascular necrosis).

After 3 months most hips are normal and X-rays show a good acetabular roof. If at 12 months the femoral head is still not correctly placed, rotation osteotomy is performed.

Hydrocephalus Diagnosed when the head circumference increases too rapidly. When hydrocephalus is likely, as in spina bifida, head circumference is measured every day. CT scan is performed to exclude subdural haemorrhage and a ventriculo-atrial or ventriculo-peritoneal shunt is inserted. The latter are better as they are longer, need changing less frequently and a blocked lower end requires only a minor abdominal operation.

Microcephaly This is suspected from the infant's appearance (small forehead) and confirmed by a head circumference below the third centile. The baby is always severely mentally impaired. A CT scan is usually performed. The parents need specialist genetic counselling but it is necessary to exclude other causes of a small head:
– congenital infections (CMV, toxoplasma)
– craniostenosis (fused sutures requiring surgery)

Note: Rarely, a reduced BPD can be due to bicornuate uterus and this can mimic microcephaly for some weeks.

Cleft lip and palate The lip is repaired by about 6 months and the palate at 12 months. The parents can be reassured that the results are excellent and should be shown photographs of successful repairs. A baby with a cleft palate may need to be fed by a spoon or with a specially long teat, but breastfeeding is often possible. A dental plate may be fitted early to allow effective sucking. Parents should join the Cleft Lip and Palate Association. There is a 1 in 20 chance of a second affected child (1 in 10 if a parent also has it).

Congenital heart disease Approximately 8 in 1000 live children are born with congenital heart disease but only 1 or 2 will present with life-threatening symptoms. Presentation within the first week or two of life is often related to closure of the ductus arteriosus. Babies present with cyanosis or heart failure:
1. *Cyanosis*
   – transposition of the great arteries
   – pulmonary atresia $\pm$ VSD
   – tetralogy of Fallot
   – critical pulmonary stenosis
2. *Heart failure*
   – coarctation
   – hypoplastic left heart syndrome
   – critical aortic valve stenosis

Prostaglandin infusions restore and maintain the patency of the duct. Detailed echocardiography will reveal the structural abnormality.

Referral to a paediatric cardiology centre for assessment and/or early surgery may be required.

Infants with asymptomatic murmurs should be assessed in an out-patient setting.

Oesophageal atresia

90%   A blind oesophageal pouch above and a tracheo-oesophageal fistula (TOF) which connects the trachea and lower oesophagus (hence there is gas in the stomach)

7%   No fistula (no gas in the stomach)

3%   H-fistula (but no atresia) – cyanotic episodes on feeding and recurrent chest infections

Suspected from:

   ultrasound scan in utero

– previous hydramnios

– frothy secretions at the mouth

– cyanotic attacks

– mild abdominal distension

It should always be diagnosed *before* the first feed, which will cause aspiration and choking. Pass a nasogastric tube into the stomach and check for acid aspirate. A radio-opaque oesophageal tube is passed at birth if there was hydramnios, and if atresia is suspected an X-ray is taken. The tube is aspirated every few minutes to keep the upper pouch clear until the infant reaches a specialised surgical unit.

Direct anastomosis is performed and the baby is fed by gastrostomy until it is healed. Gastro-oesophageal reflux commonly occurs and requires medical and/or surgical treatment.

Anorectal malformations

The anus may be displaced or may be imperforate due to:

– simple membrane

– absent anus + fistula (to vagina, urethra or skin)

– absent rectum + fistula (to vagina, urethra or skin)

Rarely, there is no fistula and there is intestinal obstruction. At 24 hours of age, a lateral abdominal X-ray is taken with the baby inverted and a metal marker on the anus. The position of the terminal gas bubble distinguishes between low (anal) and high (rectal) lesions.

Anal deformities can be corrected by local surgery 1 or 2 days after birth. The puborectalis ensures continence.

Rectal deformities are difficult to correct. A high sigmoid colostomy is performed and the definitive pull-through operation is delayed until 6 months to decrease the operative mortality. Associated abnormalities include renal, cardiovascular, high gut atresias and sacral anomalies.

Talipes

Twice as common in boys. 30% are bilateral. The foot points down and the heel faces inwards. If the deformity can be over-corrected by gentle manipulation, it is postural (due to uterine pressure). The mother is taught to dorsiflex the foot at the time of each feed and it returns to normal in 2–3 weeks.

If the foot cannot be dorsiflexed fully, then the problem is structural and orthopaedic referral is necessary. Strapping is used from day 2 to hold the foot dorsiflexed, and this is replaced weekly. Severe cases may be operated on at 3–6 weeks.

Talipes may be associated with neurological problems.

◆ Examination of the newborn

The neonate is often examined the day after delivery to reassure the parents. However, examination around day 7 is also important because VSD murmurs tend to appear some time in the first week, as pulmonary pressures fall. CDH is also easier to diagnose with certainty after a few days, when normal hips are less lax.

1. *Check the history* (drugs or illness in pregnancy, hydramnios, gestation and birth weight, labour and delivery, any family history of abnormalities). Most of the examination relies on careful observation.

2. *General appearance.* It is important to observe general movements, tone and reactions. Floppiness can be associated with Down's syndrome. The mother should be present as she often needs reassurance about common skin blemishes (see below). The normal baby is pale pink and often has slight peripheral cyanosis. Note any:
   – pallor (?anaemia, spleen)
   – plethora (polycythemia)
   – jaundice
   – central cyanosis (tongue, lips)
   – pustules (?staphylococcal infection)

3. *Face.* Note micrognathia (the infant has to be nursed prone to prevent the tongue occluding the airway) or low-set ears (associated with renal and other abnormalities). Down's syndrome is suggested by slanted palpebral fissures, marked epicanthic folds, small mouth, protuberant tongue, flat occiput and palpable third fontanelle.

4. *Head.* Measure head circumference, palpate the anterior fontanelle for tension and assess the baby's alertness and symmetry of movements. Exclude a midline dermal sinus between the root of the nose and the occiput.

5. *Eyes.* Holding the baby up and gently swinging round usually causes the eyes to open. Exclude:
   – congenital cataract
   – congenital glaucoma
   – coloboma
   – conjunctivitis (gonococcal, chlamydial)

6. *Mouth.* Examine with a torch for:
   – cleft palate (palpate also)
   – candidiasis
   – natal teeth
   – cysts (gum or floor of the mouth – excised if large)

7. *Neck.* Goitre is usually obvious. The small hole of a branchial sinus, however, is often first spotted by the mother. Redundant skinfolds on the neck can occur in Down's syndrome but are marked in Turner's syndrome (with widely-spaced nipples and lymphoedema of the legs).

8. *Chest*. There should be no intercostal recession and the respiration rate should be below 50/minute. If these signs are abnormal, chest X-ray is indicated. Breath sounds are not helpful.
9. *Murmur*.
   a) A mid-systolic murmur in a well baby is usually due to a persistent ductus which closes around day 7. Observe.
   b) A loud systolic murmur or one that persists after day 7 is usually due to VSD or pulmonary stenosis. Palpate the femoral arteries to exclude coarctation. CXR and ECG are needed.
   c) A murmur with heart failure (poor feeding, tachypnoea, large liver) indicates coarctation or multiple cardiac defects (usually transposition or hypoplastic left heart) and needs urgent referral for echocardiography and surgical correction where possible.
10. *Abdomen*. Liver, both kidneys and sometimes spleen are palpable but should not be enlarged. A palpable bladder in a boy suggests urethral valves. Examine the umbilicus for infection, discharge (persistent urachus) or herniated mesenteric duct (resembling a polyp). Inspect the anus for patency and position.
11. *Genitalia*. A hooded prepuce suggests hypospadias (refer to a surgeon). Check that the testes are descended. In a girl exclude labial fusion or clitoral enlargement.
12. *Limbs and spine*. Check:
    – hips for dislocation
    – feet for talipes
    – hands and feet for polydactyly
    – spine for midline pit (above S2 it usually communicates with the theca)
    These problems need referral to orthopaedic surgeon, plastic surgeon or neurosurgeon.

◆ Harmless anomalies

Some harmless things that the mother may need reassurance about are:
1. Subconjunctival haemorrhage. These disappear in 2–3 weeks.
2. Epithelial pearls (white spots) commonly occur on the hard palate. Disappear in 2–3 weeks.
3. A short lingual frenulum needs no treatment and never affects speech.
4. 'Sucking calluses' on lips. In fact these crusty folds can occur in babies who have never sucked. They may be shed and others reform.
5. Watering eye due to a blocked tear duct. This usually resolves spontaneously. If it persists beyond a year, refer to an ophthalmologist who may probe the duct.
6. Breast engorgement. Commonly occurs in male and female infants. They may lactate ('witch's milk'). It can last for several weeks and the parents should be advised not to try to squeeze the milk out because this may introduce infection. Spreading erythema suggests mastitis, which requires treatment with antibiotics. If an abscess forms it must be drained.

7. Umbilical hernia is common, particularly in West Indian babies and is rarely due to cretinism. It is gone by the age of 3–6 years and surgery is rarely needed.

8. Early urine may stain the nappy pink because it contains urates. This is harmless.

9. Small hydroceles are common. They are usually gone in 4–6 weeks and need no treatment.

10. Vaginal discharge or bleeding can occur around day 4 due to maternal hormones that crossed the placenta. It is harmless.

◆ Skin blemishes

- erythema neonatorum
- stork marks
- erythema toxicum
- milia
- sudamina
- strawberry naevus
- Mongolian blue spot
- port wine stain

1. *Erythema neonatorum* is a brilliant lobster-red flush that often develops all over the body. It fades within 24 hours and must not be mistaken for infection. During the first few days a line of demarcation may occur in the midline, the *harlequin colour change*, which is a harmless vasomotor phenomenon.

2. *Stork marks* (capillary haemangiomas) are present in 50% of babies, usually on the face or back of the neck. They blanch on pressure. Most fade away spontaneously.

3. *Erythema toxicum* (neonatal urticaria) is only seen in term babies and affects about 30%. It usually appears by day 2, is gone by day 7, and the baby remains well. It is possibly a histamine effect following contact with clothing, since it rarely affects the face, palms or soles. The lesions are red blotches, sometimes with white vesicles (eosinophils) in the middle. If these are marked with a ring it can be demonstrated that they fade after a few hours and others reform.

4. *Milia* are tiny papules ('millet seeds') on the cheeks and nose that are commonly seen in the first few days. At a first glance they often look as if some talcum powder has been left on the baby's face. They are due to blocked sebaceous ducts and fade in 1–2 weeks.

5. *Sudamina* is a rash of vesicles, usually on the forehead, that can develop in the second week. It is due to blocked sweat ducts and is more common in hot weather.

6. *Strawberry naevus* (cavernous haemangioma) is a conspicuous lesion that usually develops around 4–6 weeks. Strawberry naevi can occur anywhere, and large facial ones can be quite disfiguring. They increase in size in the first 6 months, then regress, and most are completely gone by the age of 7 years. They tend to bleed easily on minor trauma, and can become infected. Parents may need a lot of reassurance that they do regress.

7. *A Mongolian blue spot* occurs in 5% of white and 90% of coloured babies. It is a grey–blue discoloration, usually in the lumbar region but sometimes over the whole back. It may be mistaken for bruising. It fades within 2 years.

8. *A port wine stain* (capillary naevus) is a developmental dilatation of capillaries, usually on the face but it can occur anywhere. It is permanent and does not blanch on pressure. In the *Sturge–Weber syndrome* a capillary naevus in the distribution of the first two divisions of the trigeminal nerve is associated with a vascular malformation of the underlying cerebral hemisphere that restricts its growth and becomes calcified.

◆ Undescended testes

The testes normally descend around 36 weeks gestation. In 20% of premature male infants and in 2% of term male infants one or both testes are still undescended. *In many cases they descend during the first months, but never after a year.*

If the testicle cannot be stroked down to be 4 cm below the pubic tubercle it is maldescended. It cannot be retractile until the cremasteric reflex develops at 4–6 weeks and then flexing the hip on that side or a warm bath will bring it down.

The child is referred to a surgeon for *orchidopexy*, usually performed at about 4 years. Spermatogenesis can be irreversibly impaired after the age of 6 years and the undescended testis is 30 times more likely to undergo malignant change. 10% have an associated hernia, in which case herniotomy and orchidopexy are performed as early as possible.

Bilateral undescended testes, particularly with hypospadias, suggest that the child may be a masculinised female, and chromosomal analysis is indicated.

◆ Circumcision

Mothers are often worried that the meatus in the foreskin is too small: by pulling it distally the slit can be demonstrated easily. No attempt should be made to retract the foreskin until the child is about 4 years old because of the mucosal damage which can occur, with later adhesions and the need for circumcision.

Circumcision is a religious requirement for Jews on day 8 and in Moslems between 3 and 15 years. Even in Britain, 10% of boys are circumcised by the age of 1 year. It is contraindicated if there is hypospadias, as the prepuce is needed for repair. The only medical indications are *recurrent balanitis* or a narrow opening in the foreskin (*phimosis*) causing 'ballooning' at the beginning of micturition.

◆ Routine care of the newborn

1. At birth the nasopharynx is cleared. A soft tube can be passed down the oesophagus to exclude atresia and to aspirate amniotic fluid from the stomach, if there is meconium-stained liquor or

after delivery by section. A plastic, crushing *Hollister clamp*, which does not come loose as the cord shrinks, is put on the cord about 2.5 cm from its base.

2. *Vitamin K* (oral or i.m.) can be given soon after birth. One in 400 babies develop haemorrhagic disease of the newborn (because it takes the gut flora that produce vitamin K two weeks to become established).

   Some units give vitamin K routinely; others reserve it for 'at risk' babies, e.g. preterm, forceps or difficult delivery. Intramuscular vitamin K has been implicated in the development of childhood tumours, although further studies have failed to confirm this association. Intramuscular vitamin K is more effective than oral vitamin K, especially in the breastfed baby.

3. The baby is given straight to the mother who is encouraged to put the baby to the breast. Bottle-fed babies should be offered a feed within 4 hours of birth. The baby should be in a cot next to the mother, unless he has to go to the SCBU.

4. Immediately after birth the infant is examined for congenital abnormalities or birth trauma. Almost all serious abnormalities in neonates are apparent within 48 hours. If an abnormality is found, a nurse should be present when the mother is told, so they can discuss it later. The midwife usually assesses the Apgar score at 1, 5 and 10 minutes, weighs the baby, measures its length and head circumference, takes a rectal temperature, puts a plastic identification band on the wrist and checks that there are three placental vessels (two suggests a renal anomaly).

5. The full routine examination of the neonate is performed by the houseman the day after delivery or before discharge. The mother should be present so she can discuss any problems (see skin blemishes and harmless anomalies).

6. Vernix is wiped off the baby's face at birth but otherwise this is left to flake off. The baby is *bathed* once on the day of discharge. The normal newborn sleeps most of the time between feeds, crying if hungry, thirsty or in pain.

7. *Dextrostix* measurements are important, 8-hourly for 48 hours, if the baby is liable to hypoglycaemia (i.e. is small-for-dates or the mother was diabetic). Significant hypoglycaemia in a neonate is a level below 2.5 mmol/l.

8. *The cord* is kept dry and clean with chlorhexidine in spirit daily. It usually separates around day 7 and then takes 3–4 days to granulate over. It must be inspected daily for signs of infection, and this is one reason why the district midwife visits daily after discharge.

9. The midwife charts the weight and temperature and inspects skin, eyes, mouth (for thrush) and umbilicus daily. The rectal temperature should not drop below 36 °C. Weight loss occurs for the first 4 days and birth weight is regained by about day 10. Eye drops or swabs are no longer used routinely. Regular observation is important and any discharge is swabbed for culture. Gonococcal conjunctivitis (now rare) can blind and is notifiable. Chlamydia should be sought even in the presence of gonococcal infection as the two may coexist.

10. *Urine* is often passed soon after delivery and may be dark or pink at first. Pressure on the bladder may stimulate micturition, but no urine by 24 hours in a boy suggests urethral valves. Sticky, dark green *meconium* is normally passed within a few hours of delivery and is often preceded by a white plug of mucus. No meconium passed by 48 hours suggests intestinal obstruction. The stools become more liquid and yellow after 3 or 4 days of milk.

11. *The Guthrie test* is performed routinely on day 7, after 6 days of milk feeds. Capillary blood is taken from a heel prick and tested for phenylalanine. If phenylalanine levels are high, due to phenylketonuria, a low phenylalanine diet can prevent brain damage. All areas now screen for TSH or T4 on the same sample to detect hypothyroidism.

◆ Nappy rash

- ammoniacal dermatitis
- seborrhoeic dermatitis
- frequent loose stools
- candidiasis
- contact sensitivity (washing powder)

1. *Ammoniacal dermatitis* is caused by the wearing of continually damp nappies (faecal bacteria break down the urea to produce ammonia). Erythema and erosion appear. It soon heals if left exposed. Otherwise, advise changing napkins regularly, using napkin liners and applying a protective cream (zinc or silicone) at each change. If it has not healed within a week there is usually a secondary infection with *Candida*, or contact sensitivity (rinse nappies thoroughly).

2. *Seborrhoeic dermatitis* always begins before the age of 3 months and is gone by 9 months. It is a badly named rash characterised by erythema and scaling in the napkin area and also affecting the neck, face and scalp (cradle cap). There is no itching or soreness. Characteristically the baby remains well. The rash clears within a few weeks with 1% hydrocortisone. Crusts on the scalp can be removed with 0.5% salicylic acid in soft paraffin (left on the scalp for an hour, then removed with shampoo). Again, secondary infection with bacteria or *Candida* is common.

3. *Peri-anal excoriation* is usually due to diarrhoea and frequent acid stools. Expose and protect with zinc cream.

4. *Candidiasis* is fiery red with a scaly margin and satellite lesions. Treat with oral nystatin and nystatin cream at every nappy change. Check for *Candida* in the baby's mouth or the mother's breast.

◆ Bottlefeeding

There is little to choose between the various brands of milk for normal babies, and the common habit of running the gamut to find the one which suits the baby is illogical. Cow's milk preparations are 'humanised' and mimic human milk by being low in protein, high in lactose and low in solute. They are fortified with vitamins and iron.

Hospitals now use pre-packed sterilised feeds. Once at home, the mother has to learn how to measure out scoops of a dried powder formula and mistakes are common. The bottle and teats should be kept in dilute hypochlorite (Milton). If bottles are made up early they should be kept in the fridge and re-warmed before use. Undiluted cow's milk (doorstep milk) is too concentrated and should not be used before 10 months.

The first feed is given as early as possible after birth. The baby needs 150 ml/kg/day ($2\frac{1}{2}$ oz/lb/day). The amount given is increased (to mimic breastfeeding) from 20 ml/kg on day 1 to 40 ml/kg on day 2, etc., so that 150 ml/kg is reached by day 7.

Note: 1 oz = 30 ml = 30 g is a useful equation when discussing feeds with non-metric mothers.

The baby is fed every 3–4 hours at first, missing out the night feed after a few weeks. The regime should be flexible, because all babies are different (150 ml/kg/day is a guide) and the baby can usually be fed to satisfy his appetite. A baby that is crying may be thirsty rather than hungry. Premature babies need relatively more, e.g. 200 ml/kg/day.

Allergy to cow's milk protein can occur, causing diarrhoea and colic. There may be a family history of atopy. The baby may have a peri-oral rash. Experimentally, blood mixed with milk produces high levels of histamine. The baby can be fed on a soya-based milk.

◆ Breastfeeding

Compared with cow's milk, human milk has:
- *more lactose*, and therefore (since human milk is isosmolar) less solute. This makes the gut contents more acidic and hence more bactericidal
- *less protein*, and a ratio of casein to lactalbumin of 1 : 1 (cow's milk is 4 : 1), making it more easily absorbed
- *the same quantity of fat*, but with a higher level of polyunsaturated fats, which are possibly essential and the fat is more easily absorbed
- possible *bactericidal factors*: IgA, lysozyme, lymphocytes, lactoferrin and prostaglandins. The gut contents of breastfed babies are virtually sterile and they never get gastroenteritis. The first colostrum is particularly rich in IgA

Advantages
1. It is the ideal way to promote bonding.
2. The fat and protein content are ideal and better absorbed (and possibly vary as the child grows). Obesity is rarely a problem in breastfed babies.
3. Suckling stimulates oxytocin release and speeds up involution of the uterus (the after-pains of feeding).
4. No danger of gastroenteritis.
5. Less danger of cow's milk protein allergy (and possibly eczema). For this reason, if complementary feeds are necessary, a pre-digested milk can be used (e.g. Pregestimil).

Problems that used to be associated with bottle-feeding, however, obesity, hypernatraemia and hypocalcaemia (high phosphates binding calcium)), are now uncommon with the low-solute humanised preparations.

Physiology

1. Colostrum appears from 28 weeks and consequently the nipples should be washed regularly in later pregnancy because blocked lactiferous ducts predispose to later breast engorgement.
2. The high levels of oestrogen in pregnancy inhibit prolactin secretion, but after these fall milk secretion starts (hence engorgement tends to occur, around day 4). Nipple stimulation also causes prolactin secretion.
3. Suckling causes oxytocin release and contraction of the myoepithelial cells (and uterus) and milk let-down. This reflex is strongly influenced by higher centres, and the baby's cry can cause milk let-down. Conversely, if the mother feels anxious or nervous, milk let-down can be completely inhibited.

   Spurts of milk can occur, due to this reflex, but this does not mean that there is necessarily a lot of milk available.
4. The *best stimuli for milk production* are:
   - frequent suckling
   - breast emptying

   Therefore, if there is insufficient milk the baby should be put to the breast more frequently and the breasts should be expressed after each feed to ensure that they are completely empty.

   A high fluid intake is totally unnecessary – starving mothers can produce adequate breastmilk. Each breast produces about 50 ml per feed.

General advice

1. Start breastfeeding in the labour ward. Babies are often reluctant to take the nipple at first and the mother may need encouragement to persist. The baby should have its neck slightly extended and the whole nipple well inside his mouth.
2. There should be no restriction in the duration or frequency of feeds and babies should not be switched between breasts after an arbitrary time.
3. Demand feeding helps bonding and improves milk-flow.
4. Express the breasts after each feed to improve milk-flow.
5. Colostrum is secreted for 2 days, then milk starts to appear. If the baby is hungry, encourage suckling. Give 5% dextrose before resorting to complementary milk feeds. A well-hydrated baby can manage on little milk, certainly for the first 5 days.
6. The stools in breastfed babies can be green and very frequent (e.g. hourly) when abundant milk starts to flow, around day 5, but characteristically they become less frequent, and by 4 weeks may only occur every few days (one more advantage of breastfeeding!).
7. It is advised to give breastfed babies 5 drops per day of children's vitamin drops until the age of 2 years.

◆ Feeding problems

1. *Poor weight gain.* The baby loses weight for about 4 days (up to 10% of birth weight), regains his birth weight by about day 10 and

then gains about 30 g a day for the first 4 months ('an ounce a day except on Sundays').

Plotting a growth chart is the best way to assess adequate intake but, as a guide, the baby should double its birth weight by 5 months. If growth is poor he needs larger and more frequent feeds.

2. *Air swallowing* can cause possetting (regurgitating milk) and may be caused by the hole in the teat being too small or too large. Thickening the feeds can sometimes reduce troublesome regurgitation.

Sometimes gulping occurs if breast milk let-down is rapid, especially on the first feed of the day. Adequate winding is advised, and if this problem is very troublesome, the first 30 ml can be expressed and re-fed later.

3. *Hunger.* The baby may seem continually hungry; he may just be thirsty, especially in hot weather, and need extra water rather than milk; he may not be getting enough milk and the mother's method of making up feeds should be checked; he may just be greedy.

4. *Insufficient milk.* Breastfed babies sometimes get insufficient milk without complaining and they can develop dark green stools with mucus (starvation stools).

The amount of breast milk the baby is getting can be worked out by test-weighing him before and after each feed. If increased suckling and expressing does not increase the supply, complementary feeds or a change to bottle-feeding may be necessary. (Test-weighing has to be carried out over 24 hours to be accurate, and often causes maternal anxiety.)

5. *Cracked nipples, engorgement, mastitis, breast abscess and drugs* – see section on the breast in Chapter 4.

6. *Reluctance to feed* may be due to oral thrush or a blocked nose, but *can* be a sign of severe illness.

◆ The low birth weight baby

About 7% of all babies weigh 2.5 kg or less at birth and are defined as low birth weight (LBW). About two-thirds of these are preterm and one-third are small-for-dates.

90% of LBW babies spend some time in SCBU and babies under 1.5 kg may spend 3 or more months there. Babies under 750 g or of less than 26 weeks gestation are unlikely to survive.

Neonatal intensive care may involve:
- biochemical monitoring
- umbilical artery catheterisation (for gases)
- mechanical ventilation
- total parenteral feeding
- drug therapy (mainly antibiotics)

Vitamin supplements (e.g. Abidec 0.6 ml daily) are given from the fourth week to the age of 2 years. Iron supplements are started once the baby is 4 weeks and continued for 6 months.

Regional SCBUs have definitely lowered the mortality rate (by about 2 per 1000). There has also been a dramatic reduction in cerebral palsy (diplegia, hemiplegia and quadriplegia) in LBW babies. However, long-term follow-up studies of LBW babies that survive their stay in SCBU are needed. Preliminary reports suggest that poor bonding, slow development and clumsiness are more common.

◆ The preterm infant

The preterm infant is defined as a baby of <37 weeks gestation. More than 90% of those born at 32 weeks now survive. Of the very preterm, only 6% survive at 23 weeks (see Table 8). The cause of premature labour is usually unknown. Compared with the SFD baby, the preterm is less at risk during labour and delivery but is *especially vulnerable during the neonatal period due to immaturity of organ systems*.

Features: The baby has a feeble cry and a characteristic appearance with thin, red, shiny skin, lanugo, no vernix, a relatively large head, a protuberant abdomen and the legs lie in a frog position due to poor tone. The clitoris appears large and intersex may be mistakenly suspected. The testes may be undescended.

Problems: The baby has poor temperature regulation, poor sucking, swallowing and breathing reflexes and a tendency to apnoeic attacks. He therefore needs to be nursed in an incubator on an apnoea mattress, and tube-fed via a nasogastric tube. The other *problems* are:
– RDS (occurs in 50% under 32 weeks)
– jaundice (immature liver enzyme systems)
– intraventricular haemorrhage (delicate vessels)
– infection (immature immune system)
– hypoglycaemia

Table 8 Outcome for extremely premature infants

Gestation (weeks)	Survival (%)	Survival without handicap (%)
<23	6	50
24	26	50
25	43	50
26	60	60
27	70	70
28	80	80
29	90	90

The recognition that low birth weight was sometimes due to IUGR rather than prematurity was a landmark in perinatal medicine.

◆ The small-for-dates (SFD) infant

The baby's weight is below the 5th centile (for that population) for his gestational age. The gestation estimated by dates and scan can be confirmed (± 2 weeks) by a detailed neurological and physical examination of the baby.

Causes: Growth retardation is usually due to placental insufficiency, but the baby may be small due to congenital abnormality (10%) or infection (CMV, rubella) and these must be excluded.

Features: The baby is usually thin and long, with wrinkled skin due to protein-energy deprivation, and has meconium staining of skin, nails and cord due to fetal distress. Such babies are often pink, due to polycythemia (PCV > 70), secondary to intrauterine hypoxia. Unless ill, they feed competently and experience little physiological weight loss.

Note: This classic picture is rare now due to fetal monitoring.

Problems: The growth-retarded fetus has an increased chance of intrauterine or intrapartum asphyxia. Hypoxia causes the passage of meconium and fetal gasping, hence the tendency to meconium aspiration. There is an increased neonatal mortality rate due to:
– meconium aspiration
– hypoglycaemia (decreased hepatic glycogen)
– polycythemia (jaundice, thrombosis)
– hypothermia (loss of subcutaneous fat)

Management includes aspiration of meconium from the trachea under direct vision at birth, gastric aspiration to prevent the meconium aspiration syndrome and 8-hourly Dextrostix for 3 days.

◆ Neonatal jaundice

The danger of neonatal jaundice is that the high levels of unconjugated bilirubin can cause kernicterus (when the baby becomes irritable and hypertonic) with subsequent retardation, spasticity and high-tone deafness.

Any severely jaundiced infant must have serial bilirubin estimation. An increased fluid intake and phototherapy control the serum bilirubin level in most cases. If the bilirubin rises above 350 μmol/l (20 mg/dl) exchange transfusion may be necessary. The danger level is lower if the infant is preterm, or if hypoxia, asphyxia or hypoalbuminaemia is present (e.g. a sick premature baby would have an exchange transfusion above 200 μmol/l).

The time of development of neonatal jaundice is dependent on its pathogenesis:

day 1   – haemolytic
day 2–3 – physiological
day 4   – infection
day 10   – prolonged

Haemolytic jaundice   This develops early because the placenta no longer removes bilirubin. Any baby that is jaundiced on day 1 must be tested for:
– Hb
– group (mother and infant)
– Coombs' test
– serial bilirubins

Coombs'-positive haemolysis is due to Rhesus incompatibility or, more commonly, ABO incompatibility (mother O, baby A) which is usually mild. (Coombs'-negative haemolysis is due to spherocytosis or G6PD deficiency, but these usually present after day 1.)

Physiological jaundice

This condition affects 50% of babies and is due to low glucuronyl transferase levels. It develops on day 2 or 3, peaks around day 5, does not rise above 200 µmol/l and is gone by day 10. The baby is completely well.

Bilirubin may rise dangerously high, however, if the baby is preterm or if red cell breakdown is increased (e.g. polycythemia, extensive bruising, cephalhaematoma). *Admit if unwell* or bilirubin is above 250 µmol/l (15 mg/dl) on a dermal icterometer.

Infection

Infection, especially a UTI, must be excluded if jaundice develops after day 3 or if the baby becomes unwell:
- MSU
- blood cultures
- chest X-ray
- lumbar puncture
- swabs (umbilicus, throat, stools)

Prolonged jaundice

Prolonged jaundice (after day 10) in a well baby who is entirely breast-fed is usually *breast milk jaundice*. It can last for several weeks. It is harmless and, provided the baby is well, can be ignored. Always exclude *hypothyroidism*, which classically presents with prolonged jaundice (TSH is often screened by the Guthrie test). In prolonged jaundice caused by the following conditions the baby is usually unwell:
- UTI
- galactosaemia (urine clinitest positive)
- spherocytosis (splenomegaly)
- biliary atresia (steatorrhoea)

Send blood for a blood count, bilirubin (conjugated and unconjugated) and α1-antitrypsin levels, and urine for culture and reducing substances.

Hepatitis (due to rubella, CMV, toxoplasmosis, α1-antitrypsin deficiency or idiopathic) and *biliary atresia* both cause a raised conjugated bilirubin (hence there is no danger of kernicterus) with deep jaundice and pale stools, usually developing around the third week. A hepatobiliary scan, liver biopsy, laparotomy and cholangiogram may be needed to differentiate them. It is essential to diagnose biliary atresia by 2 months of age if a Kasai procedure is to be successful.

◆ Vomiting

- regurgitation (a feeding problem)
- infection
- intestinal obstruction
- pyloric stenosis
- raised ICP
- CAH
- hiatus hernia
- NEC

1. *Regurgitation.* Most babies regurgitate some milk and air after feeds ('*possetting*'). This can be troublesome if the baby swallows a lot of air with the feeds. This may be due to the hole in the teat being too small or too rapid initial let-down from the breast, poor attachment to the breast or simply to a greedy baby. Adequate winding and larger or more frequent feeds may be required.
2. *Infection* must be excluded in any baby who is vomiting (MSU, swabs, blood cultures, LP). If diarrhoea develops, the diagnosis is probably gastroenteritis.
3. *Intestinal obstruction.* Any baby with *bile-stained vomiting* has intestinal obstruction and should see a surgeon within the hour. There is usually abdominal distension. An inguinal hernia can strangulate easily in the neonatal period and is easily overlooked. *Always examine the groins of a vomiting baby.*
4. *Pyloric stenosis* usually presents between 3 and 6 weeks but can present earlier. Diagnosed by a test feed, i.e. feeling for a pyloric 'tumour' (like the tip of the nose) during a feed. Treated by pyloromyotomy under local or general anaesthesia.
5. *Raised ICP.* Ultrasound or CT scans may be necessary if irritability, drowsiness, tense fontanelle or fits suggest *cerebral* or *subdural haemorrhage*. Subdural haematomas can be tapped.
6. *The adrenogenital syndrome* is suspected by virilisation in girls, but in boys it presents around day 7 with vomiting. There is hyponatraemia and serum potassium is high (usually low in vomiting). It is diagnosed by a raised serum 17-OH progesterone level. It is treated with cortisone. It is essential to make a firm diagnosis before starting steroids.
7. *Hiatus hernia* is diagnosed by a barium swallow after the above causes are excluded. The baby is nursed head-up on a tilted surface.
8. *Necrotising enterocolitis* (NEC) is classically seen in preterm infants with an umbilical artery catheter, but can occur rarely in term infants. Mesenteric thrombosis causes gut necrosis and secondary infection, with abdominal distension, vomiting and melaena. Abdominal X-ray shows air in the gut wall. Treatment involves i.v. fluids, antibiotics and bowel resection. Mortality is 22%.

Haemorrhagic disease of the newborn can cause *bloodstained vomiting*, usually between days 2 and 4 – 1 mg of vitamin K i.m. is given immediately and blood is transfused. There may also be some blood in the vomit in:
– tube feeding
– cracked nipple (maternal Hb)
– hiatus hernia

In summary, a detailed history is often diagnostic, but the following may be necessary:
– infection screen
– U&E
– test feed
– abdominal X-ray
– barium swallow
– ultrasound or CT scan

◆ Diarrhoea

- gastroenteritis
- infection (UTI, septicaemia)
- drugs (antibiotics, iron)
- (rare: cystic fibrosis, thyrotoxicosis, CAH)

Diarrhoea means frequent watery stools (that may even be mistaken for urine). Dangerous *dehydration can occur within hours*. Signs of dehydration are: loss of turgor, sunken eyes and fontanelle, no urine for 6 hours and weight loss.

Breastfed infants may pass loose green stools with mucus every hour or so at first, as lactation becomes established around day 4–5, but they 'never' get gastroenteritis.

Management
1. Barrier nurse. Stools can be sent for electron microscopy (85% due to rotavirus) and culture (15% due to *E. coli*). Urine should also be sent for culture.
2. Stop milk unless breastfed, and give 150 ml/kg per 24 hours of glucose-electrolyte mixture (e.g. Dioralyte) for 24 hours. Hourly feeds can be tried if there is only occasional vomiting. Once the diarrhoea is controlled, milk is gradually re-introduced. *Drugs such as kaolin or Lomotil are unnecessary and can be dangerous.*
3. If there is persistent vomiting, the baby has to be admitted for i.v. fluids and U&E monitoring. Admit also if dehydrated or diarrhoea relapses.
4. Recurrence of diarrhoea is usually due to too rapid reintroduction of milk feeds, but may be due to secondary *lactose intolerance*, when the stools are Clinitest-positive. It can be confirmed by sending the stools for sugar chromatography. Lactose-free milk may be necessary for several months (e.g. Nutramigen).
5. *Having excluded other causes, the possibility of cow's milk allergy* is usually considered, and the baby tried on a soya-based preparation.

◆ Constipation

Provided there is no difficulty or distress in passing a stool, *the frequency of defaecation is not important*. Some breastfed babies only pass a stool every 4–5 days. If the stool is hard and painful, increasing the baby's water intake or adding half a teaspoon of sugar to each feed may suffice. If not, a daily glycerine suppository will soften the stool. In severe persistent constipation consider:
- Hirschsprung's disease
- hypothyroidism
- hypercalcaemia
- polyuria (diabetes insipidus, renal tubular acidosis, salt-losing CAH)

◆ Dyspnoea

- RDS
- pneumonia (±aspiration)
- pneumothorax

- diaphragmatic hernia
- congenital lobar emphysema
- pulmonary hypoplasia
- choanal stenosis
- congenital heart disease
- severe anaemia

Most of the above can be differentiated on a CXR.

Pneumonia is likely if the membranes were ruptured for more than 24 hours. It may follow meconium aspiration or, in a preterm baby, aspiration of regurgitated milk.

Tension pneumothorax requires a chest drain and should be suspected in any baby that 'goes off'. Small, asymptomatic pneumothoraces are not uncommon in babies for a few days after delivery.

Diaphragmatic hernia large enough to present as dyspnoea requires immediate gastric aspiration, endotracheal intubation and urgent repair.

Congenital lobar emphysema (very rare) is over-distension of one lobe caused by an abnormal bronchus acting as a valve and requires urgent lobectomy.

Pulmonary hypoplasia is associated with oligohydramnios which may, for example, be caused by renal agenesis, obstructive uropathy, or prolonged rupture of membranes. Oligohydramnios and/or renal abnormalities may be suspected from antenatal scans. Prognosis is poor.

Choanal stenosis is posterior nasal obstruction. The baby has a submandibular recession as it tries to mouth-breathe, and an oropharyngeal airway produces immediate relief.

Congenital heart disease. A large liver or weight gain suggests heart disease, and an ECG is necessary. If the baby is pale, check the Hb, as a blood transfusion may be life-saving.

◆ Respiratory distress syndrome (RDS)

RDS is likely to occur if the L:S ratio is below 2. It is due to deficient surfactant. It affects 50% of babies under 27 weeks gestation and is more common in infants of diabetic mothers. The incidence and severity have been greatly reduced by the use of antenatal steroids in premature labour. The *signs* appear within 3 hours of birth:

- tachypnoea
- recession
- expiratory grunt
- cyanosis (later)

CXR may show a ground-glass appearance with an air bronchogram, but its main use is to exclude other causes of dyspnoea.

Management
1. Oxygen given by continuous positive airways pressure (CPAP) via a nasal prong, face mask or endotracheal tube. The CPAP prevents collapse of the alveoli.
2. Oxygen is monitored by transcutaneous oxygen electrode, or pulse oximeter, and kept between 6.7 and 12.0 kPa (retinopathy of prematurity).

3. Ventilation is needed if the pO_2 falls despite CPAP, if the pCO_2 rises or if apnoeic attacks develop. There is a tendency now to early ventilation, especially for LBW babies.
4. Fluid balance is monitored. A metabolic acidosis can occur due to poor perfusion and boluses of colloid may be necessary.
5. Intravenous fluids may be needed for severe dyspnoea, but often the baby can be fed via nasogastric tube.
6. Antibiotics are given because the differentiation of RDS and pneumonia (especially that due to group B streptococci) can be difficult.
7. Surfactant derived from artificial or animal sources, given into the trachea, has greatly improved the clinical course for babies with RDS (40% reduction in mortality).

◆ Convulsions

– hypoglycaemia
– hypocalcaemia
– meningitis
– cerebral oedema (or haemorrhage)

1. Suck out the pharynx, lay the baby on his side, give oxygen, and if still fitting give phenobarbitone 10 mg/kg i.v. followed by a further 10 mg/kg 30 minutes later if no response.
2. Dextrostix. Hypoglycaemia – defined as blood glucose of <2.2 mmol/l – can cause brain damage. If suspected, take blood for glucose and give i.v. 10% dextrose (4–6 ml/kg), followed by continuous 10% dextrose infusion.
3. If plasma calcium is below 1.8 mmol/l with a normal Dextrostix, then give 10% calcium gluconate 0.2–0.5 ml/kg i.v. over 15 minutes or until seizures cease.
4. If glucose and calcium are normal, meningitis must be excluded.
5. Phenobarbitone is given if fits follow birth asphyxia and trauma. Ultrasound may be indicated to diagnose intracranial haemorrhage.

◆ Hypothermia

Hypothermia is a persistent rectal temperature below 35°C and can be fatal. It still occurs in the newborn, especially in LBW babies discharged home to poor conditions in cold weather. The *signs* are:
– weak cry
– poor sucking
– slow reaction to handling
– cold, red skin
– twitching
– oedema (hands and feet)
– sclerema (hardening of subcutaneous tissue)

It may cause hypoglycaemia, uraemia, cerebral damage and death.
The baby should be admitted in an incubator for re-warming and biochemical monitoring.
In a cold environment, bonnet, bootees and mittens will help a term infant to retain heat, but a small baby with a low metabolic capacity needs an environmental temperature of at least 27°C (80°F).

6. The DRCOG exam

The examination regulations changed following a review in 1993: make sure you have the up-to-date regulations from the College. Contact:

The Examination Secretary
Royal College of Obstetricians and Gynaecologists
27 Sussex Place
Regents Park
LONDON NW1 4RG
Tel: 020 7772 6200
Website: www.rcog.org.uk
E-mail: Coll.Sec@rcog.org.uk

◆ Key entry requirements (as at March 2000)

Always read the latest requirements for the exam you intend to sit. The exam regulations booklet includes the syllabus you should cover.

1. Must be entered as a fully registered practitioner in GMC register or Medical Council of Ireland. Date of entry must be given and a copy of the current certificate of registration submitted.
2. Apply on the approved RCOG form
   – deadline for April exam is 1st February
   – deadline for October exam is 1st August
3. Entry fee payable in sterling with application (check amount with Exam Secretary). Payment by cheque to 'Royal College of Obstetricians and Gynaecologists'.
4. Candidates must complete a recognised combined appointment for six consecutive months. It is not essential to complete this training by the time of the examination. However, successful candidates will be required to provide a certificate confirming the completion of six months of recognised training at the time of applying for registration as a Diplomate of the College.

   In special circumstances part-time training in recognised posts is permitted provided College approval is obtained in advance.

   The training posts for the exam must be held in the UK or the Republic of Ireland.

◆ The exam itself

The syllabus is largely straightforward as the exam is orientated towards the clinical aspects of the subject most relevant to GP practice. The best time to sit the exam is therefore towards the end of your Obstetrics and Gynaecology job(s) or soon afterwards, when your knowledge is up to date and fresh in your mind. The examiners are chosen from current Obstetrics and Gynaecology consultants (often

RCOG tutors) from teaching and district general hospitals, and a large numer of practising GP principals also examine. You may not be examined by a consultant or GP with whom you have worked, or who is otherwise known to you. The exam is held on a single day twice a year (on a Saturday) in April and October: several UK centres participate.

The exam is in two parts with a break for lunch in between. Some candidates will do the MCQ first while the others do the OSCE, swapping for the afternoon session.

The Multiple Choice Questions (MCQ) paper (2 hours)

There are 60 five-part questions. There is no negative marking so you should answer *all* the questions. Marking is done by a computer – follow the instructions carefully to ensure your paper can be read by the scanner. Read each section of the question carefully – highlighting key words in the question helps focus the mind on what *is* being asked, not *what you think is* being asked.

The Objective Structured Clinical Examination (OSCE) paper

There are 22 stations, with 6 minutes allocated for each station. Of these, 2 are rest stations, 15 are factual question sheets, and 5 are interactive stations. The OSCE examinations lasts approximately 2 hours and 15 minutes.

You will be given a pack with named blank answer sheets: make sure it is *your* name and that you are not scoring marks for someone else! Although they are very carefully checked, do check you are using the appropriate number sheet for each station before writing your answers. Place each completed sheet in the basket for collection as you move to the next station.

Is casual dress OK? – yes for the MCQs, but remember that in the OSCE session you will be meeting role players and having mini-vivas so it is probably better to look (and feel) the part for that half of the exam. There's no need to go over the top – comfortable and smart is the ideal.

The rest stations

These stations are there in order for you to gather your thoughts, but your previous station sheets will have been collected already so *you may not use this time to correct or revise any of your previous answers.* As they are interspersed between the other stations you may find yourself starting the OSCE session at a rest station: don't be put off. At the rest station, don't go over in your mind what you have already done – it cannot be changed now. Look around the room quickly to get a feel for where the interactive stations are. This will help you settle at them more quickly. Stay calm!

The interactive stations

These are of two types:
1. Two stations are usually with the examiner alone – a bit like a viva – they will tell you what topic you will be discussing with them and question you. To make sure it is fair for everyone, there

are 'crib sheets' for examiners to make sure that they cover a specific range of issues in that topic with you. You will score a mark if you correctly answer in each of those areas. Listen carefully to make sure you are clear what they want. Be concise (but not abrupt) to score most points.

2. The other stations will each have one or two examiners plus a role player – often a medical student – who will be assuming the role of a patient (or perhaps a relative) in a given clinical situation. *A reserve role player and sometimes reserve examiners sit at each station too – ignore them.* On the desk will be a short typed paragraph for you to read. This explains the scenario, so read it quickly but accurately. Take a deep breath and begin your interview *with the role player,* not the examiner! *The examiners are observing only and may not prompt or quiz you: concentrate on the role player.* The station is marked on set criteria: a possible 8 marks are awarded by the examiner on factual content and 2 given by the role player on what they thought of your interview skills, manner etc. and whether they would be happy to see you as their doctor again. Putting the patient at ease, appropriate eye contact, lack of medical jargon, ability to explain the issues clearly, and covering all the key points will score most marks.

The written stations Consist of several part- or mini-questions (the topics on any one sheet are related): the maximum mark is 10 for each station. These written papers are marked centrally by teams of examiners at the RCOG on the day after the exam. Each answer you give will be awarded 1 or 0 mark according to model answers agreed by the examiners. *It is therefore hugely important to read the questions carefully.* Remember that writing two paragraphs for one part-question will not score you any more than a single correct word or a well-chosen sentence giving an accurate and full answer. Never write *nothing*!

◆ Revision and exam technique

1. Always write or say *something*: there is no negative marking. Write legibly.
2. **READ** THE QUESTION – READ **THE** QUESTION – READ THE **QUESTION** ... ! This might seem obvious, but examiners are repeatedly amazed by the number of people who obviously haven't read the question *properly*. Here are some examples of impossible-looking (but still all too commonly seen) errors:
   – If the question asks *'What are the components of one ampoule (1 ml) of X?'*, the answer must be something whose total volume is 1 ml, not '500 mls of A and 10 mls of B'
   – If the question asks *'For what reason is substance Y given prophylactically in the labour ward?'* the answer should not be: 'to *treat* Jones' disease' *(0 marks)*. It would be better (but still partly wrong) if you write: 'to *prevent* the onset of Jones' disease' *(perhaps 1 mark)* and absolutely perfect if you write: 'to *prevent the mother/ baby* getting *Smith's* syndrome' *(2 marks)*.

- If the question asks *'Name one non-surgical approach useful in the treatment of heavy periods',* the answer *cannot* be: 'trans-cervical resection of the endometrium' but *could* be: 'non-steroidal anti-inflammatory drugs' or 'cyclical progestogens'.

Reading these three examples, you will all be thinking that you could not possibly make such errors yourself. People do, every year. Ensure that *you* do not, by READING THE QUESTION.

3. You will not get maximum points by repeating yourself. *Make the most of what you know.*

   If the question asks: *'Give two complications which occur more commonly in multiple pregnancies'* you will score only one mark for:
   - (1) high blood pressure, (2) pre-eclampsia
   - (1) haemorrhage, (2) PPH

   You would get two marks for:
   - (1) preterm labour, (2) pre-eclampsia
   - (1) haemorrhage, (2) malpresentation

   However, each OSCE station is marked in isolation so, although examiners don't often test the same thing twice, the same facts *may* be appropriate on more than one answer sheet.

4. *Neonatology.* You might not have done any paediatrics. Take time to learn a bit about blood gases, hypoglycaemia and resuscitation. Read through your local hospital's guidelines on the neonatal problems you might see on a postnatal ward, the follow-up arrangements for neonates who have been in SCBU, and the rules on contraindications to infant vaccinations.

5. *Brush up on your visual diagnostic skills.* There are often pho-tographs relating to a question. Microbiology is an area many people get stuck on – go back to a basic text, especially the microscopy appearance if it is classical. Also use photographic or colour atlas/picture diagnosis books for practice.

6. *Practise.* There are good sample MCQ questions around and OSCE techniques and examples are covered in some of the books.

7. Think about what you have been doing on the wards for the last 6 months, not what you read last night.

Further reading

◆ General reading

Balen AH, Smith JH 1992 The CTG in Practice. Churchill Livingstone, Edinburgh

Gibb D 1991 A Practical Guide to Labour Management. Blackwell Scientific Publications, Oxford

Hoghton M, Hogston P 1991 MCQs for the DRCOG. Churchill Livingstone, Edinburgh

Lewis TLT, Chamberlain GVP 1990 Gynaecology by Ten Teachers, 15th edn. Edward Arnold, London

Lewis TLT, Chamberlain GVP 1990 Obstetrics by Ten Teachers, 15th edn. Edward Arnold, London

Loudon N, Glasier A, Gebbie A (eds) 1995 Handbook of Family Planning and Reproductive Health Care, 3rd edn. Churchill Livingstone, Edinburgh

Reports on Confidential Enquiries into Maternal Deaths in the United Kingdom. Triennial Publications by HMSO, London

Roberton NRC 1993 A Manual of Neonatal Intensive Care, 3rd edn. Edward Arnold, London

Slade R, Laird E, Benyon G (eds) 1993 Key Topics in Obstetrics and Gynaecology. BIOS Scientific Publishers Ltd, Oxford

Studd J (ed) Progress in Obstetrics and Gynaecology. Churchill Livingstone, Edinburgh (series – considerable detail, more for MRCOG, but worth dipping into on certain topics)

◆ Worth keeping in your surgery

Chamberlain GVP (ed) 1992 How to Avoid Medico-Legal Problems in Obstetrics and Gynaecology. RCOG, London

Guillebaud J 1993 Contraception: Your Questions Answered, 2nd edn. Churchill Livingstone, Edinburgh

Guillebaud J 1993 The Pill: Your Questions Answered, Oxford University Press, Oxford

Redman C, Walker 1992 Pre-Eclampsia – The Facts. Oxford Medical Publications, Oxford

Whitehead M, Godfree V 1990 HRT: Your Questions Answered. Churchill Livingstone, Edinburgh

Glossary of abbreviations

ACTH	Adrenocorticotrophin
AFP	Alphafetoprotein
AID	Artificial insemination by donor
AIDS	Acquired immune deficiency syndrome
AIH	Artificial insemination by husband
ALT	Alanine transaminase
AP	Anteroposterior
APH	Antepartum haemorrhage
APTT	Activated partial thromboplastin time
ARC	AIDS-related complex; Antenatal Results and Choices
ARM	Artificial rupture of (fetal) membranes
ASD	Atrial septal defect
AST	Aspartate aminotransferase
b.d.	Twice a day (*bis in die*)
BMI	Body mass index
BP	Blood pressure
BPD	Biparietal diameter
BRCA	Breast cancer gene
BSE	Bovine spongiform encephalopathy
BSO	Bilateral salpingo-oophorectomy
BTBV	Beat-to-beat variation
BTC	Basal temperature chart
CA125	Cancer antigen 125
CAH	Congenital adrenal hyperplasia
CDH	Congenital dislocation of the hips
CESDI	Confidential Enquiries into Stillbirths and Deaths in Infancy
CF	Cystic fibrosis
CIN	Cervical intraepithelial neoplasia
CLASP	Collaborative Low Dose Aspirin in Pregnancy (study)
CMO	Chief medical officer
CMV	Cytomegalovirus
CNS	Central nervous system
CPAP	Continuous positive airways pressure
C/S	Caesarean section
CSF	Cerebrospinal fluid
CT	Computerised tomography
CTG	Cardiotocograph
CVA	Cerebrovascular accident
CVP	Central venous pressure
CXR	Chest X-ray
D&C	Dilatation & curettage
DGH	District General Hospital
DHEAS	Dehydroepiandrosterone
DIC	Disseminated intravascular coagulation
DRCOG	Diploma of the Royal College of Obstetricians and Gynaecologists
DVT	Deep vein thrombosis

ECG	Electrocardiogram
EDD	Estimated date of delivery
ERPC	Evacuation of retained products of conception
ESR	Erythrocyte sedimentation rate
ET	Embryo transfer
EUA	Examination under anaesthetic
FBC	Full blood count
FBS	Fetal blood sample
FDA	Food and Drug Administration
FDP	Fibrin degradation products
FH	Fetal heart; family history
FHA	Family Health Authority
FNA	Fine needle aspiration
FPA	Family Planning Authority
FSE	Fetal scalp electrode
FSH	Follicle stimulating hormone
FTA	Fluorescent treponemal antibody (test)
FTI	Free thyroxine index
FU	Follow-up
GA	General anaesthetic
GFR	Glomerular filtration rate
GIFT	Gamete intrafallopian transfer
GLT	Glucose load test
GnRH	Gonadotrophin releasing hormone
GP	General practitioner
GPI	General paralysis of the insane
GTT	Glucose tolerance test
GU	Genitourinary
Hb	Haemoglobin
HC/AC	Head circumference/abdominal circumference
HCG	Human chorionic gonadotrophin
HDL	High density lipoprotein
HFEA	Human Fertilisation and Embryology Authority
HIV	Human immunodeficiency virus
HPF	High power field
HPL	Human placental lactogen
HPV	Human papillomavirus
HRT	Hormone replacement therapy
HSV	Herpes simplex virus
HVH	Herpes virus hominis
HVS	High vaginal swab
ICP	Intracranial pressure
ICSI	Intracytoplasmic sperm injection
IGT	Impaired glucose tolerance
IHD	Ischaemic heart disease
IPPV	Intermittent positive pressure ventilation
ITU	Intensive therapy unit
IUD	Intrauterine device
IUGR	Intrauterine growth retardation
IUI	Intrauterine insemination
IUS	Intrauterine system
IVC	Inferior vena cava
IVF	In-vitro fertilisation
IVU	Intravenous urogram

JCC	Joint Committee on Contraception
KPTT	Kaolin partial thromboplastin time
LBW	Low birth weight
LFT	Liver function test
LGV	Lymphogranuloma venereum
LH	Luteinising hormone
LHRH	LH releasing hormone
LMP	Last menstrual period
LOA	Left occipito-anterior
LOT	Left occipito-transverse
LP	Lumbar puncture
L : S	Lecithin : sphingomyelin (ratio)
LSCS	Lower segment caesarean section
LVF	Left ventricular failure
LVH	Left ventricular hypertrophy
MAR	Mixed antibody reaction
MCH	Mean cell haemoglobin
MCV	Mean cell volume
MOM	Multiples of the median
MRC	Medical Research Council
MRI	Magnetic resonance imaging
MSAFP	Maternal serum alphafetoprotein
MSU	Midstream specimen of urine
NBM	Nil by mouth
NEC	Necrotising enterocolitis
NND	Neonatal death
NSU	Non-specific urethritis
NTD	Neural tube defect
OA	Occipito-anterior
O/C	Oral contraceptive
OP	Occipito-posterior
PAPP-A	Pregnancy-associated plasma protein A
PCC	Postcoital contraception
PCO	Polycystic ovary syndrome
PCT	Postcoital test
PCV	Packed cell volume
PE	Pulmonary embolism
PET	Pre-eclampsia (pre-eclampsic toxaemia)
PG	Prostaglandin
PGL	Progressive generalised lymphadenopathy
PID	Pelvic inflammatory disease
PMB	Postmenopausal bleeding
PMS	Premenstrual syndrome
PNM	Perinatal mortality
POD	Pouch of Douglas
POH	Past obstetric history
POP	Progesterone-only pill
PPH	Postpartum haemorrhage
PPS	Postpartum sterilisation
PR	Per rectal (examination)
p.r.	per rectum (prescription)
PS	Pulmonary stenosis
PV	Per vaginam (examination)

215

p.v.	per vaginam (prescription)
q.d.s.	Four times a day (*quater die summendum*)
RBC	Red blood cell
RCGP	Royal College of General Practitioners
RCM	Royal College of Midwives
RCOG	Royal College of Obstetricians and Gynaecologists
RCPCH	Royal College of Paediatrics and Child Health
RCT	Randomised controlled trial
RDS	Respiratory distress syndrome
RIF	Right iliac fossa
RPOC	Retained products of conception
RTA	Road traffic accident
SB	Stillbirth
SBE	Subacute bacterial endocarditis
SCBU	Special care baby unit
SCJ	Squamo-columnar junction
SERM	Selective (o)estrogen receptor modulator
SFD	Small-for-dates
SHBG	Sex hormone binding globulin
SHO	Senior house officer
SIDS	Sudden infant death syndrome
SLE	Systemic lupus erythematosis
SROM	Spontaneous rupture of the membranes
SSRI	Selective serotonin re-uptake inhibitor
STD	Sexually transmitted disease
SVC	Superior vena cava
TAH	Total abdominal hysterectomy
TB	Tuberculosis
TCRE	Transcervical resection of endometrium
t.d.s.	Three times a day (*ter die summendum*)
TIA	Transient ischaemic attack
TIBC	Total iron binding capacity
TOF	Tracheo-oesophageal fistula
TOP	Termination of pregnancy
TPHA	*Treponema pallidum* haemagglutination (test)
TPI	*Treponema pallidum* immobilisation
TPR	Temperature, pulse, respiration
TSH	Thyroid stimulating hormone
TUR	Transurethral resection
TURP	Transurethral resection of the prostate
U&E	Urea and electrolytes
USS	Ultrasound scan
UTI	Urinary tract infection
VDRL	Venereal Diseases Research Laboratory (test)
VE	Vaginal examination
VIN	Vulval intraepithelial neoplasia
VLDL	Very low density lipoprotein
VMA	Valinylmandelic acid
VSD	Ventricular septal defect
WBC	White blood cell
WHO	World Health Organization
YS	Year survival (e.g. 5-YS)

Index